For Pet's Sake, Do Something!

Book Two:
How to Heal Your Sick, Overfed
And Bored Pets with Nutrition,
Supplements, Herbs and Exercise

Dr. Monica Diedrich

For Pet's Sake, Do Something!

Book Two:
How to Heal Your Sick, Overfed
And Bored Pets with Nutrition,
Supplements, Herbs and Exercise

ISBN 9798884759596

Published by:
Two Paws Up Press, P.O. Box 6107
Anaheim, CA 92816-6107
Email: drmonica@petcommunicator.com
Website: http://www.petcommunicator.com

Table of Contents

Table of Contents (cont'd.)

Epilogue

About the Author

Acknowledgments

Writing a book is a very interesting process.

As an author, you begin with a heartfelt dream. In this series, it's about how to make the world a better place for pets. You want to empower others with the information they need to improve the quality of their pets' lives. You're confident you *can* make this dream come true.

You begin by assembling your research and recording your thoughts. Your dreams weave their magic as you carefully prepare each chapter. The day dawns when you feel as if you're almost finished.

Then, it happens. You discover you're not even close. Before it will ever be ready to print, the manuscript still needs considerable re-shaping and polishing. That's why we need editors.

These are the "people beneath our wings," the ones who help us arrange our thoughts, correct our grammar, and assist in conveying all of the important ideas we want to share.

In the process of working together, your editor becomes your sounding board, your constant e-mail partner, and if you're very lucky, your friend.

In 2004, when I thought my second book was publication-ready, I was truly blessed to re-connect with a former client who soon became both my primary editor *and* friend. She patiently reviewed the manuscript, showed me what still needed to be done, and willingly volunteered to do it.

Colleen Fox is that special person. Together, we've worked almost as one spirit. Her uncanny ability to put my thoughts—and my heart—into words never ceases to amaze me.

She's given me the benefit of her knowledge, wisdom and expertise and has helped me bring my second, third and fourth books through the writing and editing process. We'll soon be finishing my fifth book together (the third in this series).

For the countless hours she's devoted to making my dreams a reality, her willingness to meet unexpected deadlines, and the consistent quality of her work, I owe her unending gratitude.

Also, a special thank you goes to Paul McNeese for formatting my work into a finished book design and for shepherding the book through the publication process. His technical expertise has been invaluable.

Along the way, there've been several very knowledgeable people who've offered helpful recommendations. For sharing both their expertise and encouragement, I'm especially grateful to Dr. Robert E. Woods, DVM, Marie Cargill, Susy Guerra, Nancy Allah, Ellen Atkins, and Kathleen Widdison and her husband.

Colleen and I are also very grateful to Karen Burgess. It was just two weeks before a major deadline when the hard drive on Colleen's computer failed completely. Karen provided the uninterrupted use of her laptop for several days so work on the manuscript could continue during repairs. Her gracious gesture prevented what would otherwise have been a major setback.

And finally, I send my special love and gratitude to Chop Chop, my beloved Shih Tzu friend and teacher. He crossed over The Rainbow Bridge on February 22, 2006 at almost 14 years of age. Many years ago, he asked me to *"Do something"* when he was very young and almost at the point of death. His request helped to save his life then, and it soon became the inspiration for me to write this series of books to show others how they can *"Do something,"* too.

Introduction

When I was writing my second book *Pets Have Feelings Too!*, I knew that I also needed to write a third book. This one would be a "how to" guide for everyone who wants to do all they can to help their pets, especially when they're in distress of any kind.

After doing only a little research, though, I realized that all of the information I wanted to include was far too much to be contained in a single volume. What began as an idea for a third book has now become a multi-book series. All three of these books are based on the principle that *you* can *"Do something."*

I first learned the importance of *doing something* myself many years ago when my two year old Shih Tzu, Chop Chop, was in such distress that he seemed about to die. Two veterinarians had confirmed that there was nothing else they could do to help him. I knew his time was very short, even possibly only a matter of hours.

As I lay next to him on the floor feeling utterly hopeless, I heard him say to me, as clear as day: "You call yourself a healer. You've helped a lot of people. *So do something!"* His words played over and over in my mind until I finally realized that there *was* something I could do. The only option I seemed to have at that moment was to use spiritual healing. I began treatments right away. Chop Chop's recovery was practically miraculous, and he lived a healthy, happy life until he was almost fourteen. It was his admonition to me that inspired me to share a multitude of practical techniques with you so that you, too, can *"Do something"* for your own pets.

You can learn how to communicate with your pets and also read about a variety of useful spiritual healing methods in the first book of this series *For Pet's Sake Do Something -- How To Communicate With Your Pets and Help Them Heal.* But for most of us, we need to actively *"Do something"* on a daily basis to provide optimal health for our pets, or help them overcome health challenges that aren't life threatening. That's what the second and third books in this series are meant to help you do.

For those of you who haven't yet read any of my first three books, let me take a moment to share some of my background with you.

Since the age of eight, I've been able to understand what animals are trying to tell us. They "talk" by sending us pictures, something I call picture telepathy. You, too, can understand this kind of communication if you're able to quiet the chatter of your own mind long enough to receive the picture impressions your pet is trying to send you.

For me, this natural ability has truly been a gift. When I was young, I often tried to "turn it off" because my family and friends didn't understand it. They sometimes laughed at me, or even ridiculed me. But in my late teens, I began to nuture and use my God-given ability. It finally became apparent that my gift was leading me into the kind of work that was always meant to be my Life Assignment.

I spent several years in spiritual study, learning much more about how to use my intuitive abilities. Before long, I realized that I had a very deep love for helping animals express themselves, and helping them and their humans better understand each other. From that time on, I devoted myself to working exclusively with pets.

But as an animal communicator and spiritual healer, how did I reach the point of writing a book about nutrition, herbs, supplements and exercise?

I've always had a sense that high quality nutrition is very important for both humans and pets. Over the years, from the time I was a teenager, I made it a point to read everything I could about the subject. And because I love pets so much, I've always been alert to new ideas and products that can improve the quality of their health.

Growing up in Argentina, after I became aware of my intuitive gift, I learned from our neighbors' dogs how very much they liked to eat fruits and vegetables. They'd find them on the ground, pick them directly off the trees, or relish them as leftovers from people. They also told me that cheese was one of their favorite delicacies, and drinking cows' milk, still warm in the bucket, was a special treat. Cats said they enjoyed eating raw liver, stomach and other parts of cows, pigs and sheep. Eventually, I realized that all of these animals were eating whole natural foods, or foods from other animals. They were eating much like animals living in the wild do, because we didn't have commercial pet foods available the way we do today.

Then a number of years ago, in my work as an animal communicator, I went to talk to two West Highland White Terriers, Casey and Peaches. Their mom, Colleen, has since become my primary editor. I was intrigued by the high quality nutritional supplements she was giving to both of her dogs. What I learned on that visit sparked my interest to study even more about the many nutritious foods and healing remedies available for our pets.

By the time I decided to write this series of books, I'd already discovered an incredibly wide variety of healing modalities we could use, but nowhere could I read about all of them together in a single book, or even in a series of books. That became my motivation to compile all of this information in one place, or at least in one series. It's meant for those readers who want to learn about the multitude of methods we can use to help our pets regain their health, or simply enjoy greater health and vitality on a daily basis.

In this second book of the series, *For Pet's Sake, Do Something! – How To Heal Your Sick, Overfed and Bored Pets With Nutrition, Herbs, Supplements and Exercise,* I want to show you how very important high quality nutrition is for the health of your pets, and how you can use the wonderful properties of a variety of herbs to help bring about healing for many of the problems your pets are faced with. As you'll soon see, not all pet foods are created equal.

Once commercial pet foods did become readily available, their quality was sometimes questionable. Many people have the perception that animals can eat anything, so for a long time, it seems that not much care was taken about what went into commercially manufactured pet foods.

Even substances that have been shown to have detrimental effects in humans, like chemical preservatives and dyes, were showing up more and more frequently in commercial pet foods. But these substances definitely aren't necessary in pet diets, and they're not good for them either.

Happily, nowadays, a number of pet food manufacturers have begun to use quality products and avoid those which are harmful. This is important because the saying "We are what we eat" applies to our pets just as much as it applies to people. Since it's up to you to decide which foods will provide optimum nourishment for your pets, I want to provide you with the tools you need so that you can understand the pros and cons of each ingredient in commercially prepared pet foods. If you understand what the label is telling you about these ingredients, you won't be deceived by catchy slogans or manufacturers' marketing claims.

But we'll go a big step further than that by also talking about raw natural whole food diets for our pets. I'll show you, with detailed guidelines, how to improve the nutritional quality of your pets' diets, whether you have an extremely busy schedule or plenty of time to prepare meals.

How can a raw whole food diet help a pet? One of my very early pet clients had been diagnosed with liver cancer. He was a large German shepherd who'd gone hiking with his favorite person all of his life. When he came to see me, it had become quite difficult for him to walk, and hiking was now out of the question. In fact, his favorite person thought that this might be the very day she would have to put him down.

When she brought him to see me, her dog hadn't eaten for five days. I tried giving him some raw meat, cut up in little pieces, and he ate half a pound! She couldn't believe it. Her dog lived for another year and was able to go on a two mile hike almost every day.

Although my suggestion to feed him a raw food diet did extend his life for awhile, he might have had an even longer and healthier life if he'd been started on this type of diet at an earlier age. After reading his story, you, too, may be motivated to try a natural raw food diet for your pets.

In my quest to find ways to keep our pets healthier, I've also researched a wealth of information about vitamins, minerals, enzymes and other nutritional supplements. In this book, I'll share some of my findings with you about which vitamins and minerals are beneficial or even necessary to add to your pets' meals, and why enzymes are so important. We'll also review many nutritional supplements that may help with a variety of pet health problems.

How and when you feed your pets, or when you should make major changes in their diets, are other important factors to consider, too. And besides knowing what's beneficial for your pets, it's also important to know which foods animals should stay away from, or might even be harmful to them. You'll find chapters devoted to each of these topics in this second book of the series as well.

Often when our pets have major illnesses, or some type of chronic health problem, they need to be fed a specialized type of diet. I'll share with you the results of my research about nutritional requirements for specific diseases, as well as recipes you can prepare for your own pets who have these difficult problems. But the importance of high quality nutrition is not the only topic you'll find in this book.

Usually we think of food as being something we commonly find in a grocery or pet supply store. But there's another form of food available which can be used not only as a food, but also as a "medicine."

You'll learn about how common herbs, Chinese herbs, and Ayurvedic (Indian) Herbs can add health and vitality to a pet's life, and even help your pets recover from a variety of illnesses. This section of the book also includes specific directions about how to administer herbs orally, as well as how to use them externally.

As important as high quality nutrition and herbs are for your pets' wellbeing, you'll also have much healthier, happier pets if they continue to remain physically active throughout their lives. It's not just a matter of putting your shoes on and taking your pets for a walk. There are many interesting and fun ways to provide exercise for them, both indoors and outdoors. We'll talk about some of those creative ideas, as well as jobs they can perform, in the chapter about exercise.

In your quest to keep your pets healthy, you'll find many different items you could use for their benefit, but it's neither practical nor economical to simply "buy and try." To make the decision easier about which foods, herbs or other healing modalities may be most beneficial for your pets, you'll find information in Chapter 18 about how to pre-test the items you'd like to use. This will provide you with a guideline so that you can make better choices about what you should or shouldn't give your animal friends.

My own pets have successfully benefited from a number of the remedies suggested in this book, and they've always been fed a natural whole food diet. They've lived long and healthy lives, and seldom required veterinary assistance. The same can be true for your pets.

Enjoy this second book of the series now, but be sure to watch for the third book, ***For Pet's Sake, Do Something! – How To Heal Your Pets Using Alternative Therapies.*** It will give you the opportunity to learn about healing with homeopathy, flower essences, incense, essential oils, crystals, color, sound, massage, magnets, hydrotherapy, acupressure, acupuncture and chiropractic. There will also be guidelines for using emergency first aid, and how to provide for your pets if something unexpected happens to you.

My hope is that you'll remember to go back to this series of books again and again as a reference whenever your pets experience any type of health challenge, and that you, too, will feel empowered to proactively *"Do something."* The joy you'll experience from being an active participant in your pets' healing will remain with you always.

Dr. Monica Diedrich
Anaheim, California USA
April, 2007

An Important Note
Before You Begin

In the next several chapters, I'm going to share a wide variety of information with you based on all of the research I've done. I want to provide guidelines for you so that, at a glance, you can see numerous possibilities for enhancing your pet's daily health, or for helping him or her recover from illness.

My hope in doing so is that you will then feel knowledgeable and empowered to do something positive instead of worrying and feeling helpless in the face of your pet's health challenges.

The breed of your pet, his or her weight, plus any health factors identified by your veterinarian will determine the best combination of ingredients, the amount to be used per dose or serving, and the wisdom of using any one, or a combination of, specific healing modalities you're going to be reading about.

All of these suggestions were compiled to provide you with a variety of alternative or additional treatments. *In no way do these methods replace veterinary care.* Always consult your own veterinarian, or a holistic veterinarian, who is familiar with the state of your pet's health.

And because I'm *not* speaking as a trained nutritionist or as an expert in the use of any specific kind of healing modality, I do ask that you regard this information only as a general guideline. You can then do your own research from the wealth of material which is available in books and on the internet to help you decide what may be best for your own pets.

Chapter 1

Understanding Commercial Pet Foods

Animals sometimes act just like people when it comes to eating anything and everything that tastes good to them. Just as some people will eat a whole bag of potato chips, a pint of ice cream, or a whole pie and still want more, some animals will devour a whole meatloaf, a watermelon, or the entire contents of a dinner plate or garbage bag without ever giving a single thought to how they may feel afterward, or how it may affect their well being.

But for the most part, many pets' diets are often fairly routine, sometimes even boring, and, all too often, lacking in nutritional value. When I ask most of my clients what they feed their animals, they tell me they feed "good commercial pet food and no table scraps."

My unspoken question has always been: What constitutes "good commercial pet food?" Is it good because a television ad tells us so? Or because it has a recognizable brand name or a catchy slogan? Is it good because veterinarians are convinced (usually by the manufacturer of a specific brand) that their food is the best one on the market because of all the research they've done? And how exactly do they do their research?

The truth is, pet food is only as good as the ingredients it contains, and those it doesn't, as well as how much it's been processed.

You can determine something about the quality of your pet's food by taking a moment to read the labels. Don't be fooled by the word "natural," though. Many things are natural (like sugar or fat), but they're not necessarily nutritious.

Here are some of the components of commercial pet foods you need to clearly understand.

Meal and by-products

The term "meal" appears in most pet foods, but you'll need to exercise caution when making your selection, and read those labels carefully. Some products with "meal" in them may have good nutritional value. However, others may contain ingredients you'd be very unwilling to give your pet.

A label that reads "beef, lamb, chicken, turkey, duck, menhaden fish, or any other specifically named meal" should mean that the manufacturer used *real* meat, poultry or fish sources which have been ground up into smaller pieces, or had the water extracted. The nutritional value will depend on the quality of the meat, poultry or fish used. This is generally an acceptable form of "meal" to use in your pet's diet.

On the other hand, many ingredients used in some pet foods could actually contain elements which have the potential to be harmful to the health of your pet. These are often generically identified on the label as "meat and bone meal" or as "by-products." They're the forms of "meal" that you'll most likely want to avoid using in your pet's diet.

Where do these by-products come from? Food processing plants cut away the choicest pieces of meat and poultry to be used for human consumption. Whatever is left over is often used by pet food manufacturers.

It's important to understand that these generic "meat and bone meal" or "by-products" possibly contain all of the remaining parts of a slaughtered animal. This could include bones, tissue, intestines, lungs, blood, etc.

By-products, especially from sources other than reputable food processing plants, may also include moldy, rancid or spoiled meats. Frequently, even something that starts out in good condition doesn't arrive that way because it isn't handled with proper care before it reaches the processing plant.

Some generic by-products may even come from the carcasses of dead and diseased animals. If they do, those by-products run the risk of being contaminated with cancer, pus, bacteria, hormones, antibiotics or other medications, as well as feathers, fur, flea products, and sometimes even the plastic bags containing the smaller dead animal's remains.

Why do so many pets nowadays have so many of the same diseases people do? Many reputable veterinarians have come to the conclusion that poor quality nutrition, and/or the use of potentially contaminated products, may be responsible. These factors may weaken a pet's immune system to the point that the pet then becomes unable to resist many of the diseases now commonly treated in veterinary clinics.

Good health is maintained in great part by good nutrition, so please, read pet food labels carefully. If you want pet food with a higher nutritional content, choose those products which use real meat and poultry, and possibly also contain beef, lamb, chicken, turkey or other whole food "meals," but try to avoid those foods containing potentially detrimental generic "meat and bone meals" and "by-products."

Fats

Many different types of fats may be used in the processing of pet foods. High quality pet foods use food grade oils, or oil sources like flaxseed which contain essential fatty acids (EFAs). These are part of a healthy diet. Lower quality foods will most likely use rendered animal fat, restaurant grease, or even oils which are less than fresh.

Restaurant grease consists of multiple fat sources such as butter, lard, vegetable oils, beef, lamb, poultry, pork, ham and bacon fat. It may be stored in underground vaults, or in storage containers kept outside for long periods of time where it may undergo extreme variations in temperature.

Rendering companies periodically collect this previously used restaurant grease. If the material will be used for animal feed, they treat it to remove pesticides, heat it to remove impurities, and add preservatives to the mixture to prevent deterioration. This is the mixture that pet food companies may buy and use in their products under the generic label of "animal fat." What's not sold to pet food manufacturers may then be sold for non-food uses like oil, cosmetic and skin care products, soap production or composting.

So be sure to check the label on your pet's food to be certain the types of fats used will contribute to your pet's overall health.

Additives and preservatives

Now that you know what to look for when it comes to "meals" and "fats," you then need to review the additives and preservatives in the pet food you're using.

Vitamins and minerals

Lower quality pet foods are often a combination of ingredients of variable quality and may run the risk of containing the contaminated ingredients mentioned above. Some pet food manufacturers may try to compensate for this by adding synthetic vitamins and minerals to give the *appearance* that the formula is balanced and nutritious. Usually, however, these supplements are not in addition to what's already in the food. They're being added to replace the naturally occuring vitamins and minerals that were destroyed during processing.

If those vitamins and minerals are added to high quality foods, that's a plus, but if the food sources used are of low quality to begin with, then the only real nutrients your pet may be getting aren't coming from the food itself. They're only going to be found in those added synthetic vitamins and minerals, and probably in less than adequate quantities. That might be comparable to a human eating only candy bars or fast foods for breakfast, lunch and dinner, and then taking vitamin and mineral supplements to try to make up for the lack of nutrients in the candy bars or fast foods.

Color, salt and sugar

To make food more appealing to the human eye, often a little FD&C red coloring is added. And to give it taste appeal, the mixture is seasoned with a sodium product or sweetened with a sugar product. Pets are attracted to food mostly by scent and taste. They don't need artificial colors to entice them, and they *don't* need added salt or sugar in their diets.

Preservatives

Next come the preservatives. Dry foods are usually stabilized with BHA (butylated hydroxyanisole), BHT (butylated hydroxytoluene), or ethoxiquin, all commonly used chemical preservatives that are supposed to keep food fresh "for years." And propylene glycol is often added to chewy foods to keep them moist.

In very small and infrequent amounts, these preservatives may not cause noticeable problems, but think about the quantity your pet consumes if he or she eats foods preserved with these chemicals every day, year in and year out.

Are they excreted from the body naturally, or do they build up over time? Do they put an added burden on a pet's immune system by forcing it to deal with any toxicity they may cause? Does the immune system have a double burden placed on it because it has to cope with the effects of these toxins, while having to resist other causes of disease at the same time?

Consider that these preservatives aren't ingredients found in nature, their consequences haven't been thoroughly studied in animals, and some chemical preservatives have even been shown to be potential cancer causing agents in humans.

So what kind of preservatives are acceptable? One of the most common is mixed tocopherols. Others you may see are ascorbic acid, which is a form of vitamin C, and alpha-tocopherol which is a form of vitamin E.

The moral of the story is: read the labels on your pet's food carefully. If you don't like what you see, check out other brands until you find one that has good nutritional quality for your pet.

Processing

All bagged and canned foods have been processed to some degree, but the quality of the products used, plus the method of processing, will determine how much nutritive value remains in the finished product. The more minimal the processing, the higher the nutritive value should be.

There are several processing methods used. Rendering is essentially a function of separating or processing which is used to extract oils or handle carcasses. Extrusion is a process in which heat and pressure systems "puff" dry foods into nuggets or kibbles. Baking cooks the ingredients, which in the case of grains, makes them more digestible. Each of these processes has an effect on the overall nutritive value that will, or won't, remain in the food.

However none of them will necessarily destroy the hormones used to fatten livestock or increase milk production, nor do they destroy drugs such as antibiotics or the barbiturates used to euthanize animals. This means that in the lower quality pet foods, our pets are likely to be eating food products which are still contaminated with some of these unhealthy ingredients.

What to look for in a nutshell

High quality foods will:

- Use superior sources of protein from whole, fresh meats, or use a meat meal that has been made from fresh meat
- Have a whole-meat source (like lamb or lamb meal, or chicken or chicken meal) as one of the first two ingredients, or have two meat sources listed among the first three ingredients
- Include whole, *unprocessed* grains, vegetables and other ingredients
- Use high quality food grade oils, or oils like flaxseed which contain essential fatty acids (EFA's)

- Use only preservatives like alpha or mixed tocopherols and ascorbic acid
- Have no added sugar, salt or color

You should find:

- A minimum of food fragments such as brewer's rice and wheat bran
- A minimum of meat (animal) by-products
- A minimum of processed ingredients

Lower quality foods will contain:

- "Animal protein," "poultry protein," and/or "meat and bone meal" (instead of real beef, chicken, turkey, lamb, duck, ocean whitefish or other novel and specifically named proteins)
- Animal by-products and/or poultry by-products
- Rendered animal fat, poultry fat, etc.
- Brewer's rice and wheat bran, especially among the first five or six ingredients
- Chemical preservatives including BHA, BHT, and ethoxyquin, plus propylene glycol to keep chewy foods moist
- Artificial colors and dyes
- Added salt
- Sweetners like sucrose, fructose, corn syrup
- Lots of vitamins to replace those lost in processing

* * *

The practice of good nutrition not only includes consuming the right foods and nutrients, but it also means eliminating those ingredients which could put an added burden on a pet's digestive system or immune system.

Armed with information about meals, fats, additives, preservatives and processing, you'll now be better prepared to make wise choices from the abundant variety of commercial pet foods which are available.

But there are many other wholesome ways to improve your pet's diet, too, so in the next chapter, we'll look at several alternative methods for varying or improving what your pet eats. If your pet is already experiencing health challenges, a natural whole food diet may be exactly what's needed to help overcome some of those challenges.

Chapter 2

Some Wholesome Alternatives

While there are *some* commercial dog and cat foods available nowadays which *do* provide good nutrition, there are also several alternative methods you can use if you want to feed your pet an even more wholesome diet.

Natural fresh, wholesome, unprocessed food should be part of everybody's diet—people and pets alike. Personally, I've had my own dogs on a natural whole-food diet for over twelve years, and they've been healthy, happy senior citizens who seldom require veterinary assistance or intervention.

I know it's almost impossible for you to cook for your animals regularly if you work and commute for many hours each day, but I can offer several suggestions for those of you who have even a limited amount of time to prepare something special once in awhile. And for those of you who do have extra time to devote to improving your pet's nutritional program, I'll provide some interesting options which you may also want to consider.

The three methods I'll introduce next require more preparation time than simply opening a can of moist food or a bag of kibble, yet many busy pet parents often find they can adapt one or more of these methods to work well for them.

Be good to your pets:
for the extra-busy or overworked person

Even if you regularly feed a good quality kibble, doing so may contribute to chronic disease in the long run because kibble is essentially a dehydrated product.

In Chinese medicine, dehydrated foods lead to what's called "internal heat." In time, this overloads the kidneys and the spleen. The liver also starts to heat up, and eventually your pet may experience burping, upset stomach, and throwing up bile in the morning.

To prevent the effects of using only dehydrated foods, there are a number of things even a very busy person can do.

Quick suggestions

One simple solution is to make the food wetter by adding *unsalted/unseasoned* chicken, turkey, vegetable or beef broth to your pet's kibble. This is better than using only plain water since the broth contains many nutrients, too.

Adding portions of certain types of vegetables to your pet's meal provides additional nutrition. This is easy to do when you're already preparing vegetables for yourself.

When serving your dog or cat cooked vegetables, try not to add salt or other condiments to the portion they're going to eat.

Cooked, unseasoned vegetables are fine, but *raw* vegetables are even better. Grating raw vegetables before serving them helps to make them more easily digestible.

Your dog may enjoy snacking on carrot or celery sticks during the day, and your cat may want to snack on lettuce, celery or various fruits. These can provide healthy alternative types of treats.

For dogs and cats, you can also add any kind of cooked meat to the dry food, but it shouldn't have sauces, condiments, or strong spices in it. Avoid ham, pork and bacon for both dogs and cats.

Once or twice a week, you may even want to serve a whole organic raw egg to top off a good quality dog or cat kibble. A spoonful of cottage cheese or some plain yogurt would also be a nice addition a couple of times a week.

Please be sure to study the list of **Foods All Pets Should Avoid** in Chapter 6, because there are some fruits, vegetables and other foods that *definitely should not be fed to your pet.*

Nutritional supplements

Another way to improve your pet's nutritional program is by adding supplements to the regular food you use. You might want to check out Udo's Pet Essentials for Dogs, and Udo's Pet Essentials for Cats, as well as Missing Link. These products provide food supplements, herbs, essential fatty acids, probiotics, and enzymes that aren't usually found in other pet foods. Missing Link also has a formula with glucosamine in it for seniors who may be experiencing arthritis problems.

Recipes for nutritional supplements—for dogs only

If you'd like to prepare your own blend of supplements to add to your dog's kibble, here are two recipes I've found during my research which might be helpful:

Recipe #1:

4 teaspoons vegetable oil

1 ¾ teaspoons bonemeal

50 to 200 IU Vitamin E

5,000 to 10,000 IU Vitamin A

1 lb (2 cups) ground turkey, chicken, lean ground beef, or beef heart

-----

Mix the oil, bonemeal and vitamins together. Then combine this mixture with the meat, coating it well. This yields 2 cups. Add ½ cup of this mixture to every cup of dog kibble. (If your dog normally eats less than a full cup of kibble at a time, be sure to adjust the quantity of the mixture to keep the ratio of ½ cup of supplement to one cup of kibble. To maintain a healthy weight for your pet, you may also need to reduce the amount of kibble you feed whenever you add a supplemental recipe.)

Recipe #2

2 teaspoons vegetable oil

1 teaspoon bonemeal

50 to 10,000 IU vitamin A

½ cup vegetables (raw or cooked)

1 cup creamed cottage cheese

Mix the oil with the bonemeal and vitamin A. Add the vegetables and then the cottage cheese. Add ½ cup of this mixture for every cup of kibble. (Remember to reduce the serving size, if necessary, to maintain the same ratio.)

Recipe for nutritional supplement — for cats only:

> *1 ½ cups yeast powder*
>
> *¼ cup kelp powder or ¼ cup mixed trace mineral powder*
>
> *1 cup lecithin granules*
>
> *2 cups wheat bran*
>
> *2 cups bone meal, calcium lactate or calcium gluconate (choose only one of the three)*
>
> -----
>
> *Mix ingredients together. Store in a covered container in the refrigerator. Add one teaspoon of this mixture to each of your cat's meals (twice per day). Once a week give a cat 400 units of vitamin E, 10,000 units of vitamin A and 400 units of vitamin D. Another alternative is to purchase an oil supplement for pets which contains these vitamins.*

Be extra good to your pets: cook for them once a week

The following diet can be used for both small adult dogs and senior cats, keeping a basic ratio of: 60 % protein / 20 % vegetables / 20% grains.

If you want to adapt this recipe for younger dogs and cats who have higher activity levels, you'll need to increase the amount of protein, especially for cats. A younger, very active adult dog may need as much as 70% protein, while a younger adult cat would require about 80% protein.

The measurements provided below can also be adjusted for larger breed dogs who require larger portions based on their levels of activity.

This particular recipe is not designed to meet the needs of puppies and kittens.

Select the ingredients

Choose from among the following ingredients, using one meat protein, one grain and an assortment of vegetables from the examples below for both adult dogs and senior cats:

Proteins: lamb, ground turkey, chicken or beef—all raw, and organic if possible;

Grains: brown rice, barley, millet, buckwheat or oats—in whole grain form (not instant);

Vegetables (raw): carrots, zucchini, beets, dark green leafy vegetables, parsley, garlic (in limited quantities), and alfalfa sprouts (especially for cats);

Vegetables (for light cooking): peas, broccoli, green beans; (Try to use one vegetable of each color; for instance, carrot for orange, green for zucchini, squash for yellow, etc., depending on whatever you have available that week. You may use both raw and cooked vegetables in the same meal.);

Oils: olive oil, virgin coconut oil, flaxseed oil, or safflower oil; (Avoid using corn oil and soy oil since these can be allergens. Organic Virgin coconut oil is now frequently recommended for it's numerous health benefits, but if you're using virgin coconut oil, be sure it's made only from fresh coconut meat. Avoid using any coconut oils which have been refined or purified, or have been made from dried coconut meat called copra.);

Bonemeal: You can obtain a powdered supplement with bone marrow in it from the pet store. It smells good to animals, and should be mixed in with their food. Bone meal not only has a lot of calcium in it, but it also has the right combination of calcium to phosphorous ratio. Our domesticated dog's ancestors, or wild dogs, used to eat the bone from their prey as well as eating the organs, muscles and meat. Giving our pets bonemeal instead of raw bones is a way to provide them with the benefit of the nutrients without having to worry about giving them fresh bones. Fresh *raw* bones are still preferable, but bonemeal is a good alternative, especially for those pets who have bad teeth, problems with their mouths or are just plain old and can't chew a raw bone. (Never give a pet cooked bones because they're very likely to splinter.);

Other options: tofu, lentils, kidney beans, red beans, black beans, navy beans, soybeans.

Since dogs and cats are carnivores these items are best used as supplements in addition to meat protein, not in place of meat protein.)

Prepare the brown rice

Bring 2 cups of water to a full boil. Add 1 cup of regular *brown* rice (the kind that requires cooking, not the instant variety). Cook covered for 35 minutes on low heat. Don't remove the lid for another 10 minutes after you turn off the heat. This allows the rice to absorb all the water in the pot. Then let it cool.

You may also use barley, millet, buckwheat or oats. Follow package directions for cooking any of these grains.

Prepare other ingredients

2 cups of raw vegetables (carrots, celery, zucchini, beets, green beans, alfalfa sprouts, parsley, dark green leafy vegetables, etc., and ½ clove of garlic), or slightly cook peas, green beans or broccoli (Remember, vegetables will be more digestible if they're first grated, or if you grind them using a food processor or a blender.)

2 pounds of beef, lamb, ground turkey or chicken (preferably organic)

4 teaspoons of bone meal

You can also use some tofu, which doesn't need any cooking. All beans, lentils and soybeans are also good ingredients, though they do need to be cooked first, and *soaked* before cooking so they won't cause excessive gas.

Combining and serving

You may use either of two methods:

Option 1 - (where both broth and oil will only be added to each individual serving at feeding time): Because bone meal doesn't dissolve well, first mix it in a bowl with any other powdered supplements you want to include (like acidophilus, vitamin C, kelp, etc.). Mix all of these ingredients well, then add the vegetable blend, grains and raw meat. Add unsalted/unseasoned broth (meat, chicken, turkey, or vegetable), and one type of oil, to each portion just before serving. The amount of broth you use is up to you. The entire recipe calls for 2 tablespoons of oil, so this amount should be divided among the total number of servings.

Option 2 - (add the oil to the mixture that will be frozen/refrigerated, and add only the broth at mealtime): First mix the bone meal in a bowl with any other powdered supplements you may want to include (like acidophilus, vitamin C, kelp, etc). Then add the oil and mix thoroughly making sure there is no clumping. Add the vegetable blend and the grains and mix again. Finally add the raw meat. Before you give your animal a serving, heat a little broth and mix well.

Keeping in mind that this recipe is for a small breed dog or a senior cat, separate the mixture into daily meal size servings based on your pet's breed, size and weight. If the entire portion will be used within a few days, it can be kept in the refrigerator. If you're going to serve it less frequently, the remaining portions should be frozen and defrosted when needed.

Also, use a complete daily vitamin-mineral supplement formulated for dogs or cats, not for humans. Or use one of the supplement recipes above.

Always use appropriate safety and clean up procedures for any surfaces, utensils, bowls or hands that come in contact with raw meats. If you handle raw meats, wash your hands before you touch other foods, surfaces or utensils, lest you accidentally contaminate something that might come in contact with food for people.

Be incredibly good to your pets: cook or mix every day

This is for the "*I'll do anything for my pets*" type of person.

Many holistic veterinarians recommend *raw* food, and particularly *raw* meat, as part of a regular diet for both dogs and cats. Veterinarians who believe in this diet say that feeding raw foods restores vitality, even in very sick animals, and can improve many chronic health problems. This may be due in part to the fact that live raw foods contain their own built-in supply of enzymes. Enzymes improve digestion so that vital nutrients can be more fully and abundantly absorbed by the body.

One of the most often described raw food diets is called the BARF diet (an acronym for Bones and Raw Food).

"But wait!" you're saying, "I was told never *ever* to give bones to my dog!"

That caution is correct if you're talking about *cooked* bones, because when they've been cooked, bones become dry and brittle. That's when splintering may occur, sometimes causing serious or even fatal injuries. Fresh, meaty *raw* bones, however, usually don't pose that same problem. If this is a concern for you, you can consider grinding up the bones.

"But what about the bacteria in raw meat?" you may also ask. "Isn't that harmful to a pet?"

Raw meat and bones have always been an essential part of the diets of wild animals. Our domestic pets have intestinal systems similar to dogs and cats in the wild. That's why bacteria, which may harm us as humans, doesn't affect dogs and cats in the same way.

General guidelines

Protein sources for a raw food diet

Use fresh organic meats or poultry when preparing your pet's meals. Or, check with your local pet store, since there are some companies that now provide raw foods already packaged in patties, and frozen without preservatives.

Using bones or bonemeal

A raw food diet for dogs also needs to include some meaty bones and bone marrow. Meat served alone contains phosphorus but no calcium. The bones provide the calcium necessary to balance the phosphorus in the meat. If you're not using raw, uncooked bones, then you should consider providing this balance by using a bonemeal supplement. The only bones that should be given to cats are raw chicken neck bones.

How much should you feed?

That depends on each individual pet. You need to know your pet's ideal weight and monitor it so that you can maintain it, but you'll soon find that your pet will probably eat less raw food than dry food.

As a general rule, a dog should eat an amount comparable to 2% of its body weight per day. A highly active dog or working dog may require about 3% of its body weight per day. Bear in mind that no two dogs are alike, and their age is also a major consideration. A puppy can consume up to 10% of its body weight. A cat, on the other hand, may be satisfied with about two tablespoons of fresh food per day usually divided into two servings.

Another way to look at meal planning is by counting calories. In this case, the following general guidelines would apply, but keep in mind that very active dogs and cats may need even more calories:

Daily Caloric Intake Recommendations			
Dogs		Cats	
Weight	Calories per day	Weight	Calories per day
10 pounds	410	6 pounds	191
25 pounds	840	8 pounds	255
50 pounds	1,380	10 pounds	319
70 pounds	1,690	12 pounds	383

Supplements

Also remember to add the appropriate pet-formulated vitamins and minerals to the diet to be sure it's well balanced. A holistic veterinarian can often provide the guidance you'll need to help you make the wisest choices.

Keep in mind that balanced nutrition plays a vital role in your pet's ability to think clearly, to cope with increased stress levels, and to maintain emotional balance. This is especially true of dogs who are involved in training programs. They must receive a proper balance of proteins, fats, and complex carbohydrates, as well as other nutrients, vitamins and minerals for optimum growth, general health maintenance and the repair of any damage to their immune systems. That's why supplementation is so important as part of a raw food diet.

How long can raw food be left out? When feeding raw food, if your animal doesn't eat the meat in fifteen or twenty minutes, pick it up and toss it out. Don't try to save it for later. Then clean the dish thoroughly to prevent e-coli or other bacterial contamination.

Serving raw bones: Since there may be raw meat on the bones you give your dog, you might consider feeding bones outdoors, or restricting your pet to a specific area while he or she is enjoying a meaty bone in the house. To prevent bacterial buildup in that area, you may want to be sure your dog is on a floor surface that can easily be disinfected, or on a mat that can be washed regularly. The same precautions would apply to feeding raw chicken neck bones to cats if they don't eat them directly from their bowls.

Ingredients you'll use in a raw food diet

In general, this list applies to both dogs and cats, but please note that there are several exceptions when it comes to cats.

Meats

Use fresh raw liver, kidney, brains, heart, etc. as well as fresh ground meat for both dogs and cats. Avoid using any ham, pork and bacon, however.

For dogs, *raw* meaty bones from chicken, turkey, duck, beef, lamb, venison, and bison, plus scraps such as *raw* wings, necks, backs, or carcasses may also be used.

For cats, use only raw chicken neck bones cut into small pieces. Raw chicken neck bones are round and don't splinter. About three vertebrae per serving should be sufficient. Cats can handle them easily since they're used to eating small rodents.

It's best if all of these ingredients are obtained from young animals. As animals age, they tend to absorb and store toxic materials in their bones, so logically, bones from younger food-source animals should be less toxic.

Some people grind the whole meaty bones first.

For adult dogs: Meat and raw bones with plenty of attached meat should make up 50% to 70% of their diet. The rest should be a mix of vegetables and grains.

For cats: Cats require even higher amounts of protein than dogs do. You can reduce the vegetables and grains significantly and make meat protein constitute 60 to 80% of an adult cat's diet.

Vegetables and fruits

For both dogs and cats, use fresh green leafy vegetables and root vegetables like carrots, beets, horseradish, lotus roots, parsnips, radishes, sweet potatoes, and yams, as well as certain ripened fruits. Frozen vegetables are also an alternative. If you only have canned vegetables, be sure to use the no-salt-added variety.

Pumpkin, cooked and mashed, is beneficial, too. It can help with weight loss by providing a pet with both nutrients and a sense of fullness.

Onions in any form are a no-no, and grapes should also be avoided. See the list of **Foods All Pets Should Avoid** in Chapter 6 for other fruits and vegetables that should be avoided altogether or used very sparingly for pets.

Grains

Sprouted grains like alfalfa, clover, barley, millet, etc. are used like vegetables.

Non-sprouted whole grains need to be soaked in water, juice, or milk overnight, then crushed using a food processor or juicer. They can also be ground into flour and then soaked. But for those who absolutely need the quickest method of preparation, simply cook prepared whole grains like barley, millet, oat flakes or brown rice. You can also use buckwheat, which isn't a member of the wheat family but is, instead, the fruit of a plant which is related to the sorrel and rhubarb family.

Other items to add to a raw diet for adult dogs and cats

Liver is rich in vitamins, minerals, fatty acids and protein. My research indicates that you can use raw or slightly cooked liver about twice a week. Depending on how much you use, liver will either replace another meat source, or you may choose to combine it with another meat protein to equal one serving. Be sure to use liver only from organically raised animals, otherwise the liver may be highly contaminated. And it shouldn't be fed too frequently to avoid any toxicity from the higher levels of vitamin A which liver provides.

Yogurt is excellent for tummy problems and intestinal health. Use unflavored plain low- fat natural yogurt with "live cultures," and no added sugar.

Eggs also add extra nutrition and can be used once or twice a week as long as your pet isn't allergic to eggs. Use a whole egg, egg yolk, or just the egg white. It provides nutrients for the coat and skin, is soothing to the stomach, and provides a feeling of fullness. Raw eggs (preferably organic) should always be the freshest you can find to avoid any problems with salmonella. Cooked eggs should not be seasoned or fried. (There's additional information about eggs in Chapter 6, **Foods All Pets Should Avoid.**)

Flaxseed Oil, among other remedies, is often used to treat cancer in both people and animals. It may also prove useful in the nutritional management of auto-immune diseases. Consult your veterinarian to determine the best dosage for your pet.

Mixing flaxseed oil with cottage cheese significantly increases the effectiveness of the flaxseed oil, particularly for people or pets who are fighting cancer. However, if your pet can't eat cottage cheese, feed the oil with some other type of protein to help with absorption.

It can be beneficial to add a little flaxseed oil to your pets daily meals to resolve or prevent skin problems, especially dry flaky itchy skin.

Other beneficial supplements for adult dogs and cats

I'll talk more about vitamins, minerals and supplements in other chapters, but here are some other items you may also want to use in a raw diet.

Cod liver oil, garlic, kelp powder and Vitamins B, C and E should be taken daily—or daily for a certain length of time only. Caution needs to be observed when you're using cod liver oil, garlic and oil-based vitamin E. Again, check with your veterinarian to be sure you're using the proper amount, and to determine how long a supplement can safely be used for your own pet.

Apple Cider Vinegar (brown, not white) is a good natural detoxifier for dogs and cats who have allergies, skin and coat problems, excess mucous, or are dealing with obesity. Used in a natural raw meat diet as a digestive enzyme, it may be enough for an enzyme-deficient dog or cat. You'll find much more detailed information about Apple Cider Vinegar in Chapter 4, about nutritional supplements.

For cats only

Since cats often tend to be finicky eaters, they may turn up their noses and walk away the first time you serve them a raw food diet. Don't panic. Cats like really smelly things, but sometimes a raw food mixture doesn't smell good enough to be tempting. In that case, try adding one of the following to entice them:

1. one small piece of sardine (in olive oil or tomato sauce)
2. some cooked chicken liver
3. a small quantity of baby food (experiment with sweet potatoes, creamed corn, peaches, lamb, etc.)
4. a few drops of soy sauce (sodium free)

Cats can have a very healthy coat if we add yeast, wheat bran, and kelp powder to their meals.

For cats with excessive dander, try adding lecithin granules.

Taurine is an amino acid which is absolutely essential for cats. Since they cannot manufacture it on their own, it's up to us to be sure that they receive an adequate amount each day.

Cats who are eating a fish-based diet will probably not require any supplementation.

For those cats who eat non-fish diets, clam juice is a good source of taurine, or you can give a 250 mg tablet or capsule daily, mixed in with their meals.

Also remember that cats may need vitamin E added to their diets.

For indoor cats, you'll also need to consider adding vitamin D. This vitamin is normally supplied by exposure to sunlight, so it's particularly needed in supplemental form for cats who never have the opportunity to soak up any sun on a regular basis.

For dogs and cats who are ill or recuperating

When dogs and cats are sick or for those who are recuperating from an illness or surgery, you may not be able to use a raw diet right away. As a temporary measure, you may use baby food because it's easily digestible, and it's recommended by various knowledgeable people. *Unsalted* baby mixes such as lamb, veal, turkey, rice and vegetables (without onion powder or onion salt) are great for short term usage. If you're feeding these for 5 or 6 days, you'll also need to add vitamins and minerals designed for pets to provide a balanced meal.

* * *

In the next chapter, we'll look at a variety of vitamins, minerals and enzymes that may be beneficial to use with either a commercial or a homemade diet. Also pay particular attention to Chapter 5, **Food and Water Management**, where you'll learn about several different feeding techniques, as well as how to monitor the effects of dietary changes.

Chapter 3

Vitamins, Minerals and Enzymes

Pets, like people, are individuals. They have unique nutritional needs requiring different levels of proteins, fats, carbohydrates, fiber, vitamins, minerals and other nutrients.

Even the highest quality pet foods can't fulfill the unique nutritional requirements of every individual pet, even when they're able to provide the majority of nutrients that pets need. In fact, no single food is the right food for every pet at every stage of its life. Puppies, kittens, adult dogs and cats; pets who are pregnant, lactating, older, or hard-working; and those who have medical conditions all have different nutritional requirements. Vitamin, mineral and other nutritional supplements can help meet these requirements.

All multi-vitamins for pets are not created equal, however. The vitamin supplement you give your pet should be formulated for animals, free from additives, and free from sugars. Ordinarily, a vitamin formulated for humans should not be used unless it's been veterinarian approved.

Most vitamins and minerals definitely need to be given in combination with each other because one may require another in order to do its job effectively, or too much of one may deplete another. Therefore, don't try to give a single vitamin or mineral alone just because it's ordinarily used to help a certain condition.

Make it a rule of thumb to do the research necessary to find the correct balance, and regularly consult with your veterinarian to be certain you're giving your pet what's best for him or her.

Vitamins

Vitamins are as important for our pets as they are for us because they help fortify the immune system, regulate body processes, and protect the body from environmental toxins. They also help to break down nutrients such as carbohydrates, proteins, and fats so the body can utilize them.

Vitamins work with minerals and enzymes for digestion, reproduction, muscle and bone growth, and maintenance of healthy skin and hair coat.

Vitamins are classified into two main groups: fat soluble and water soluble. Vitamins A, D, E and K are fat soluble and are retained in the fatty tissues of the body. Since the body doesn't eliminate them readily, we need to be sure we're not using excessive amounts which could cause a toxic reaction.

Vitamins B and C are water soluble. The body regularly eliminates any excess amounts of water soluble vitamins which it doesn't use. Water soluble vitamins are easily lost through processing and cooking, so your pet may need to take them in supplement form on a regular basis to get a sufficient quantity.

Vitamin A

Helps with skin problems and supports the immune system during infections. It's also essential for normal growth, night vision, and the maintenance of soft mucous tissues.

Vitamin B-Complex

Helps maintain a healthy nervous system, especially during stressful conditions. Dogs with behavioral problems or learning difficulties may have a B vitamin deficiency. Other problems which may benefit from vitamin B-Complex supplemetation may include cataracts, adrenal problems, skin allergies, skin disorders, blood vessel disease, anemia, runny eyes, slow weight gain or growth, erratic appetite, and stool eating.

In cats, the signs of vitamin B-3 or niacin deficiency are mouth ulcers, thick foul smelling saliva that drools, weight loss, lack of appetite, weakness, and apathy finally leading to death from respiratory disease. A deficiency in dogs may cause black tongue.

The B vitamins require a certain balance and should be taken together in a B-Complex formulation especially balanced for pets. If there's a reason to increase one of the B vitamins for a short period of time, it should be done with professional advice to avoid creating an imbalance that might subsequently cause other problems. Cats may require more B-Complex than dogs do.

Vitamin C

Helps strengthen the immune system because it's an anti-oxidant. Vitamin C is beneficial for the skeletal growth of large-breed dogs, for animals who are under an unusual amount of stress, and for those recovering from surgery.

Animals don't manufacture enough vitamin C on their own, so it's important to provide them with a good supplement. It's best absorbed when given with food. In humans, the ascorbate form is usually more easily absorbed and easier on the stomach than the ascorbic acid form because the ascorbate form usually has some calcium to buffer it. This may also be true for animals.

When using vitamin C, you'll know if you're giving too much if a pet develops very soft or runny stools. Use the bowel tolerance test to determine the right amount for your pet. Start with a low dose and gradually increase the amount. If the stools become loose, reduce the amount until the stools once again have normal consistency. This is true for both dogs and cats.

Vitamin D

Helps with the assimilation of calcium and phosphorus to maintain healthy bones and teeth. Indoor cats may be vitamin D deficient because they're never exposed to the sun. Though little is known about specific vitamin D requirements in animals, cod liver oil is often used to correct vitamin D deficiency. Since this is a fat soluble form of the vitamin, dosages should be professionally monitored, and given only for a specific length of time.

Vitamin E

Helps to maintain a healthy circulatory system; acts as an anti-oxidant to strengthen and protect the immune system and the lungs and defend against cancer cells; oxygenates the blood and improves the function of internal organs; may promote fertility, slow the aging process, prevent cataracts, promote skin healing, reduce scarring, relieve posterior paralysis and disc problems in dogs, reduce breast tumors, and prevent steatites (yellow fat disease) in cats. Research has proven that vitamin E also blocks arterial plaque formation which may make it beneficial for pets who are prone to heart conditions.

Vitamin K

Helps maintain normal levels of blood clotting proteins. Under normal circumstances, dogs and cats are unlikely to have a dietary deficiency of vitamin K because they manufacture this vitamin naturally in their intestines. If they have a disease in which fat is not well absorbed, then they might experience a Vitamin K deficiency.

Accidental ingestion of rodent poisons is the most common reason for vitamin K therapy in small animal practice.

Minerals

Minerals are vital for digestion, growth, and the repair of tissues. They help promote strong bones, teeth, and claws and contribute to healthy skin and hair coat.

They do this by helping the body form bone and cartilage, maintain fluid and electrolyte balance, and transport oxygen in the blood. They also help the body maintain the right acid/alkaline balance, produce horomones in the correct quantities, and keep muscles and nerves functioning properly.

Minerals work together with vitamins, enzymes and other minerals in the body to produce their effects.

Classes of minerals

Minerals are usually grouped into macro and micro categories. Greater amounts of macro-minerals are needed in the diet, and they're found in larger amounts in the body than micro-minerals.

Macro-minerals include calcium, magnesium, sodium, potassium, and phosphorus.

Micro-minerals, often called trace minerals, include a wide variety of mineral sources such as chromium, copper, iodine, iron, and manganese to name just a few. When animals lack proper amounts of trace minerals, their bodies can't function properly. This may even result in a shortened life span.

Mineral balance and supplementation

The proper balance of minerals in a pet's body is very necessary. For this reason, it's important to give a complete and balanced mineral supplement instead of giving only a few isolated minerals.

A high quality vitamin/mineral supplement will not harm a normal animal, and in many cases it will be quite beneficial. It must be specifically designed for animals, contain the proper balance of vitamins and minerals, and be given according to directions.

It's also important to understand that too much or too little of one mineral can affect the action of other vitamins and minerals in the body. Supplementing with individual minerals, or not providing one, or even several, specific minerals can create imbalances and possibly disrupt an animal's nutritional health. It's always wise to consult with an expert when it comes to vitamin/mineral supplementation.

Occasionally, it may be necessary to give more than the usual quantity of a certain mineral in order to correct a specific deficiency or excess if a pet's condition requires it, but this should only be done under the direct care of a veterinarian.

Calcium

Calcium deficiencies can result in nervousness, lameness, muscle spasm, heart palpitations, eczema, decrease in bone density, osteoporosis, gum erosion, increased cholesterol levels, seizures, hemorrhages, high blood pressure, arthritis, and bone fractures.

Care needs to be exercised when giving calcium supplements. They need to be well balanced with magnesium and other trace minerals. Too much calcium may cause kidney stones. However, adding vitamin C may prevent this from happening.

Calcium can be added to the diet in several different ways, but some are better choices than others:

1. **Bone Meal:** This comes in powder form. It's the most natural calcium source for carnivores and provides many trace minerals. It's also convenient and easy to use. It's especially beneficial for large dogs with bone problems or signs of hip dysplasia.
2. **Di-Calcium Phosphate:** This product is sometimes available in pet stores.
3. **Calcium Tablets or Powder:** Unlike bonemeal, this choice provides no additional phosphorus or other trace minerals.

If you're using bone meal, you'll notice that it doesn't dissolve easily and that it floats to the top when any liquid such as broth or water is added to it. Usually pets like the taste and smell of bonemeal, but in this state, it may have an unappealing sandy texture and taste. Instead, try mixing it in with the ground-up vegetables first, or mix it with flaxseed or olive oil. It will still be well absorbed by the body, and when it's blended in with food or oil, an animal shouldn't object to eating it.

Magnesium

Magnesium helps to detoxify the body of lead and other heavy metals. It's important for enzyme function, heart rate, bones, muscles and the nervous system. If a pet is deficient in magnesium, symptoms may include heart arrhythmias, high blood pressure, seizures, bone pain, nervousness, irritability, twitching, depression, muscle spasms and problems with weight gain. For dogs with arthritis, a calcium/magnesium supplement may be a great pain reliever.

Potassium

Deficiency symptoms of potassium include restlessness, heart arrhythmias, poor growth, muscular paralysis, tendency to dehydration, and heart or kidney lesions. Potassium helps prevent strokes. Some diuretic and heart medications deplete potassium in the body. An excellent and easy source of potassium replacement is apple cider vinegar. (You'll find much more detailed information about apple cider vinegar in **Chapter 4, Nutritional Supplements**.)

Sodium

Signs of sodium deficiency are heat exhaustion with loss of equilibrium, decreased water intake, dry skin, hair loss, retarded growth, and an inability to maintain body water balance.

Enzymes

Enzymes of various types are absolutely essential for a body to function properly. While most pets manufacture sufficient enzymes themselves, there are times when supplements may be required, particularly when it comes to helping with digestion. Enzymes are lost whenever food is cooked or processed, and their production also diminishes during the aging process.

The addition of digestive enzymes, even for healthy dogs, can help to assure that the foods and supplements they eat are broken down so that the vitamins, minerals and other nutrients will be well absorbed and used by the body. If a pet has a digestive disorder, then digestive enzymes are a must.

How can you add enzymes to a pet's diet in a natural way to help with digestion? All growing sprouts, herbs and grasses contain enzymes. The pet section of health food stores will have specially formulated products which contain a variety of greens including barley grass juice, wheat grass juice, chlorella and spirulina. Since these provide enzymes from food sources, they're particularly beneficial. In serious cases of digestive enzyme deficiency, however, your veterinarian may need to prescribe a formulation of enzymes in a higher dosage.

* * *

In the next chapter, we'll look at a wide variety of other nutritional supplements you may want to consider in order to provide the highest possible level of good nutrition for your pets, especially when they're facing health challenges.

Chapter 4

Nutritional Supplements

Nutritional supplements can be added to our pets' diets to prevent or correct a deficiency, or to enhance their overall nutritional health. Supplements come in a variety of forms such as multi-vitamins, mineral paste, fiber granules, powders, capsules, liquids, etc. They may even include healthy foods (like yogurt, eggs or cottage cheese) that aren't normally part of a pet's regular diet.

The following are some nutritional supplements you may want to consider using.

Apple Cider Vinegar (brown, not white)

. . . is rich in vitamins, minerals and potassium. It's been used to improve the health of animals from dogs to dairy cows by reducing infections, improving stamina, preventing muscle fatigue after exercising, increasing resistance to disease, and protecting against food poisoning.

It can also be helpful for reducing intestinal gas and fecal odors, relieving urinary tract infections, and alleviating constipation and some symptoms of arthritis.

It may reduce bloating after a meal or help with other digestive problems. The enzymes in apple cider vinegar may aid in the digestion of food, which in turn may help an animal who needs to gain weight.

Used as a daily supplement, it can be a good immune booster to increase a pet's resistance to disease, as well as boosting a pet's ability to recover from injuries.

A pet using apple cider vinegar may be less likely to have fleas or intestinal worms.

After exhaustion or heatstroke, apple cider vinegar can be used to restore electrolyte (sodium, potassium, chloride) balance instead of using salt.

For a dog on chemical diuretics or heart medication, it can often provide replacement of potassium that is lost through the use of those medications.

Some reference materials suggest adding a drop or two of apple cider vinegar to a pet's drinking water for general health maintenance. Others recommend adding it to food instead of water so that the water is always free from any additives, even a beneficial one.

You'll want to do your own research to determine whether or not this would be an appropriate supplement to use for your pet, and in what quantity. An easy way to do this on the Internet is to do a search using the words "apple cider vinegar for dogs" (use the quotation marks, as shown, to limit the search engine's listings).

Acidophilus

. . . are friendly bacteria which not only help with digestion, but also keep bad bacteria and excess yeast in check. They do this by restoring friendly bacteria to normal levels which then prevents the overgrowth of harmful bacteria. The use of acidophilus may also be helpful in preventing fungal growth, diverticulosis, and bad breath.

Everybody's intestines need friendly bacteria, but there are times when these helpful organisms become seriously depleted. If an animal has to have surgery or has an extended illness, the supply of the good bacteria in their intestines may be significantly reduced for a period of time.

And when an animal has to take antibiotics, the medicine doesn't discriminate between friendly and harmful bacteria. In the process of getting rid of the bad bacteria, antibiotics also kill all of the good bacteria. Taking antibiotics is sometimes a necessity, but it does create an unhealthy condition in the intestines. Since it takes the intestinal system a long time to create friendly bacteria on its own, the more effective solution is to quickly populate the body once again with lots of good bacteria. We can do this by using acidophilus supplements.

Acidophilus comes in several strains, the most common of which are lactobacillus and bifidus. A product containing multiple strains of acidophilus may be the better choice following antibiotics, while lactobacillus alone may be adequate for maintenance.

An effective way to give acidophilus to a dog is to wrap a capsule in a little bit of a high quality moist dog food, which most pets will take from your hand without hesitation.

Since I give my dogs raw food, I simply open an acidophilus capsule, mix it in with the bone meal and supplements, and then add the food. Everything needs to be mixed well to avoid clumping.

Alpha Lipoic Acid

. . . is known to improve glucose metabolism and help prevent some of the complications associated with diabetes. As a powerful antioxidant, it protects the body from the effects of free radicals, and it can be beneficial for pets who engage in very high levels of activity.

Aloe Vera

. . . has been used for centuries to relieve everything from burns to internal ailments. Some of its topical uses include treatment for rashes, sunburns, skin irritations, wounds, scarring, flea and other insect bites. Internally, it's been used to help with problems like constipation, colitis, abdominal pain, digestion, allergies, fevers, blood and lymphatic circulation, and as a support for the liver, kidneys and gall bladder.

Many people grow the plant and simply break open a leaf when they need the healing gel. However, it's important to know that when a leaf is broken, it releases an enzyme which is meant to protect the inner gel. This enzyme, when it comes in direct contact with the skin, may cause what people think is an allergic reaction. In fact, it's not an allergic reaction to the aloe vera gel; it's a reaction to the enzyme in the leaf. To avoid this problem, carefully remove the gel from the protective sheath before applying it to the skin so that the cut part of the leaf doesn't come in contact with the gel or the skin.

Another alternative is to use an aloe vera product which has been grown under optimal conditions, has been harvested properly so the enzyme doesn't get into the gel, and one in which the gel still contains all of its beneficial properties. There's a company called Aloe Life (www.aloelife.com) in Santee, California, which provides a pure aloe vera gel for pets. This formulation can be used either internally or on the skin, and it's safe for pets to lick.

Brewer's Yeast

. . . is principally grown on barley, although it's sometimes grown on molasses. It's probably best known as a by-product from brewing beers and ales, but in its healthier form, it's also grown specifically as a nutritional supplement, rich in B-vitamins, selenium, chromium, amino acids and other trace elements. There are other yeasts, known as baker's yeast and torula yeast, but neither of these provides the nutrients, especially chromium, that come from a high quality nutritional brewer's yeast.

Chlorophyll

. . . is a detoxifier and tonic. It cleanses the blood and helps to build red blood cells. Since it helps to balance blood sugar levels, it's useful for pets who have hypoglycemia or diabetes. Chlorophyll is a whole food, not a medication. It's available in powder, capsule or liquid forms and can be added to regular food or to a pet's drinking water.

CoQ10

. . . is not only an antioxidant but it's also a wonderful support for heart health. In addition, it supports blood sugar balance for pets with diabetes, and helps promote healthy gum tissue for pets with periodontal problems. As an antioxidant it can be helpful for older dogs as they age, and it provides immune boosting properties. The dose needs to be adjusted to the weight of the pet.

Essential Fatty Acids (EFAs)

. . . are required at all stages of life from infancy through old age. They may significantly lower cholesterol, benefit the circulatory system, act as an anti-inflammatory agent, strengthen the immune system, promote healthy hair and nails, and reduce cancer risks.

One essential fatty acid we and our pets usually get plenty of—even too much of—in our diets, is Omega-6. But excessively high levels of Omega-6 sometimes lead to certain health problems. What we and our pets usually need to help balance the Omega-6 is more Omega-3.

There are many products that can help pets obtain more Omega-3 in their diets. You might first consider a high quality fish oil (free from mercury), or cod liver oil (used with caution so as not to create a harmful level of excess Vitamin A). A supplement such as flaxseed oil is another option, and it's also high in beneficial fiber. Flaxseed oil can usually be found in the refrigerated section of health food stores.

It's wise to buy all of these products in the smallest quantity possible. All oils can become rancid if they're stored improperly, kept around for too long a time past their recommended expiration dates, or exposed too frequently to light and air by opening and closing the bottle many times. If you're going to buy the larger size bottle, transfer some of the contents into a smaller bottle for every day use so that the main supply is not constantly exposed to frequent periods of being open or unrefrigerated.

Evening Primrose Oil

. . . is a source of an essential fatty acid known as GLA (gamma linolenic acid). It's even considered safer and more effective than borage oil and black currant oil, both of which are also high in GLA.

Evening Primrose Oil can be helpful for preventing diabetes, promoting circulation, maintaining healthy hair, skin, and nails, and alleviating dry skin problems, skin disorders and inflammatory conditions.

When given regularly, it can help maintain a high quality coat for long coated breeds. Because it helps promote coat growth, it's invaluable to use during the molting season.

Ginger

. . . is a spice widely used since ancient times for its medicinal properties. It's beneficial for reducing nausea and helping to settle the stomach. It also helps to combat motion sickness, dispel dizziness and reduce excessive gas.

Glucosamine and Chondroitin

. . . have proven valuable for older dogs with arthritic problems. When used with calcium and magnesium, these two supplements may help prevent joint deterioration as well as strengthen overall bone health.

Kelp Powder (seaweed)

. . . is very useful for promoting good health because it's so rich in amino acids, vitamins, minerals and trace elements. It contains over 60 minerals and 21 amino acids, plus simple and complex carbohydrates and several essential plant growth hormones. It has antioxidant, antibacterial, diuretic and expectorant properties. Some Japanese research shows that it may also have anti-tumoral properties.

Lecithin

. . . is beneficial for nerve, liver, circulatory and heart health, particularly for elderly cats and dogs.

Spirulina Powder

. . . can act as a very powerful health support. In addition to providing vitamins, minerals, enzymes and trace elements, it's known for its remarkable ability to detoxify the body, regulate metabolism and help maintain a strong, healthy immune system. Spirulina works as an antioxidant, helping with the production of macrophages which, in turn, work to destroy cancer cells and other harmful organisms. It also provides some bioflavonoids and essential fatty acids.

Taurine

. . . is an amino acid which is an essential dietary nutrient for cats, especially kittens and pregnant females. However, it's something which cats cannot manufacture on their own, so they need to get it from a fish-based diet, or by being given a taurine supplement on a daily basis.

Taurine is beneficial for the brain and nervous system, and it bonds bile acids. It's also necessary for heart health in both cats and dogs. Often, a lower than acceptable taurine level is found in pets with cardiomyopathy, a disease affecting the heart muscle. This is especially true for cats, and it's also true for some larger breed dogs. For those pets with cardiomyopathy, taurine supplements, along with other supportive care, have sometimes provided beneficial effects. This may not be the case, however, if the disease is already fairly far advanced.

Cats with low levels of taurine in their diet may become blind, but the process may be reversed if it's caught within the first five months of life.

The research seems to show that low levels of taurine are often associated with a pet's diet. Some commercial pet foods may be deficient in taurine depending on how they've been processed and what ingredients they contain.

However, it's interesting to note that low levels of taurine don't occur only in pets who eat a commercially prepared diet. Even pets eating a nutritious home made diet may also show low taurine levels. In general, though, most animals will obtain enough taurine if they're fed a raw or lightly cooked meal, but cats in particular may need a supplement unless they're being fed a fish-based diet.

If you need to give your cat additional taurine, try using clam juice, or mix the contents of a 250 mg tablet or capsule in with the cat's food daily.

Liquid supplements

Why use liquid supplements? Because up to 90% of the nutrients in liquid supplements are absorbed by the body more rapidly and more completely. You may want to consider these juices not only for yourself, but also for your pet.

Most of them suggest that people take only one ounce, once or twice per day, so a bottle may last for the better part of a month. The dosage you use for your pet will depend on his or her size and weight.

Each of the liquid supplements described below is made from a unique ancient fruit that is known for its health benefits.

Noni Juice (Morinda Citrifolia)

Nobody knows for certain where the Morinda Citrifolia plant originated, but for centuries, natives of several South Pacific Islands were the only ones who knew about this plant and used it for its medicinal properties. Native Polynesians still use it to increase their vitality as well as ease pain and prevent illness.

It wasn't until around 1990 that the scientific community became aware of the many benefits which were available from the juice of this potato-sized green fruit. It's more commonly known as Noni Juice, or Tahitian Noni Juice.

As a liquid supplement with high levels of antioxidants, Noni Juice can be used to help support the immune system, the circulatory system, tissues and cells. It may also help to increase energy levels, as well as being beneficial for good digestion, because it helps the body absorb more nutrients at the cellular level. It also contains components that are important for nourishing the skin and hair.

Noni Juice seems to have almost miraculous regenerative powers in some instances, because it revitalizes the body by causing damaged cells to be renewed. The active substance in the juice, known as Xeronine, serves a vital role when it comes to cell production. If Xeronine encounters an unhealthy cell, it will encompass and enclose it, so that it can't reproduce.

All parts of the Morinda plant can be put to good use. In addition to the fruit, which is used for juice, the leaves can be used for their soothing properties, and the seeds, which are a good source of linoleic acid (an essential fatty acid), can be used to promote healthy skin.

By itself, the fruit is very tart, making it almost impossible to eat it raw, but when grape or plum juice is added to the juice of the noni fruit, it's quite palatable. It's highly recommended for all animals and humans, and you'll find it mainly in health food stores.

Mangosteen Juice

The Mangosteen fruit, known by its botanical name, Garcinia Mangostana L., is called the Queen of Fruits. It can be found in Thailand, Cambodia, Vietnam, India, the Philippines, Brazil, Africa and the Caribbean. This is a tropical fruit, about the size of a tangerine, which thrives in fertile soil and a tropical climate.

The juice of the Mangosteen fruit has two important components: beneficial antioxidants and Xanthones. Antioxidants provide support for the immune system while Xanthones have been shown to have antibiotic, antiviral, and antifungal properties as well as histamine-blocking actions.

Traditionally, Mangosteen juice has been used for multiple purposes including warding off many types of infections, protecting against disease, control of pain and fever, and increasing energy. It may also provide anti-diabetic, anti-leukemic and anti-microbial properties (to combat fungus and bacteria). Because it also appears to have anti-inflammatory properties, it may be helpful to use when skin infections are present.

While Mangosteen Juice is highly regarded for its health benefits, what first attracted the people of Southeast Asia to it was its unique sweet/tart taste. At least one website describes the juice as "good for the body—heaven for the tongue." Mangosteen Juice is available in health food stores and from independent distributors.

Berry Young Juice and NingXia Red Juice

Berry Young Juice and NingXia Red are two of the most powerful antioxidant juices on the market today. The source of their power is a small red fruit known as the Chinese NingXia wolfberry.

Both Eastern and Western scientific analyses show that the nutrient packed little wolfberry contains 18 amino acids, 21 trace minerals, 29 fatty acids, vitamins B1, B2, B6, vitamin E, plus more beta carotene than carrots, more vitamin C than oranges, and a host of antioxidant properties.

The wolfberry has an impressive list of accomplishments. It's been shown to be very useful for supporting the immune system, the liver, the kidneys, the blood, and the eyes. It's also been shown to inhibit inflammation and to have a protective effect on the cells of the pancreas which regulate the body's insulin system.

The ancient Chinese people were said to have three cherished tonics to support their health: ginseng, ling tzi, and wolfberries. Ling tzi was difficult to find, and only royalty had access to ginseng, but wolfberries were in plentiful supply, even for the common person to enjoy. Those who used them reaped wonderful health benefits and lived active lives well beyond the age of 100.

The Chinese NingXia wolfberry, which has a 5000 year history, was introduced in the United States a few years ago in Berry Young Juice, and more recently in NingXia Red Juice, both produced by Young Living Essential Oils.

Berry Young Juice uses the juice of the wolfberry, while NingXia Red uses whole-fruit wolfberry puree, which enables it to retain even more of the health giving benefits of this powerful fruit. This truly does make it one of a kind, and it has the research and the numbers behind it to support that claim.

There are several species of wolfberry, but only the most potent Chinese NingXia species is used as the main ingredient in both Berry Young and NingXia Red Juices. For those interested in using low glycemic foods, this particular species of wolfberry has a very low glycemic index of only 10.6.

This low glycemic benefit would no doubt be negated if sugary juices like pear, white grape, and apple (which don't provide high levels of health benefits) were used as sweeteners, so instead, both Berry Young Juice and NingXia Red are sweetened with organic Blue Agave.

Other healthful ingredients in both products include the juices of blueberries, pomegranets, apricots and raspberries, plus the pure essential oils of lemon and orange. Each berry, with its own impressive ORAC score, and each essential oil when used alone, provide unique nutritional support for the body, but together they provide an even more potent synergistic effect.

How do we know that? An ORAC test (Oxygen Radical Absorbance Capacity) measures how well the substances in a drink are able to neutralize harmful free radicals (substances which weaken the body's immune system and allow diseases to take over).

In independent comparison testing, both Berry Young Juice and NingXia Red Juice far exceeded other antioxidant drinks. The ORAC scores for *both* Berry Young Juice and NingXia Red were more than *double* the scores of XanGo (Mangosteen) and Noni.

NingXia Red has also been proven to absorb and neutralize four of the most prevalent free radicals, including the superoxide free radical, more effectively than even the best of other health juices are able to do.

A single ounce of Berry Young Juice or NingXia Red Juice each day can provide substantial health benefits for people. The same healthful benefits are available for pets, though the quantity given needs to be adjusted based on the size and weight of the pet.

Both the delicious Berry Young and NingXia Red juices are available through a web site, http://www.youngliving.com

* * *

In the next chapter we'll talk about several feeding techniques, as well as ways you can monitor the various effects of food and supplement changes which you may be making in your pet's diet.

Chapter 5

Food and Water Management, Plus Monitoring Dietary Changes

In addition to choosing the most nutritious foods for your pets, you also need to consider when and how to feed them in the most effective way. This varies from one animal to another. All pets in the same household shouldn't necessarily be fed the same way. It's also important to adjust the way you feed each individual pet at different stages of his or her life.

Food

General feeding guidelines

Adult dogs and cats require sufficient *nutrients* for three primary purposes: to meet their daily energy needs, support their immune systems, and repair body tissues. To obtain these nutrients, the amount of food an individual pet requires depends on the *quality* of the food, as well as on the animal's size and activity level.

You'll find manufacturer's suggestions on pet food packages about how much to feed. However, these recommendations are usually based only on a pet's weight, and in many cases, feeding that amount, plus treats, will cause an animal to put on an unhealthy number of excess pounds.

Your pet's weight should never be the only consideration when you're trying to decide how much to feed. Age, activity level, overall health, reproductive status, and the climate in which you live must all be taken into consideration to determine the amount of food your pet should consume each day. Consequently, you'll often need to decrease the quantity recommended by the pet food manufacturer in order to keep your pet's weight at a healthy level. If the recommendation on the package is a cup and a half of food per day, consider seriously that maybe this amount should be a combination of both food *and* treats.

Basic feeding formula

In general, a diet for *dogs* should consist of: *60% protein and fat, 20% vegetables, and 20% carbohydrates.*

Cats need a higher amount of protein and fat, so their formula should be: *80% protein and fat, 10% vegetables, and 10% carbohydrates.*

When feeding home cooked meals, one cup of food per day for each 25 pounds of body weight should be sufficient. If you change from a commercial pet food to a natural food diet, you'll actually see your pet begin to lose some weight. You may also notice that he eats less voraciously, doesn't drink quite as much water, and doesn't have as much urine and stool output. This is normal on a homemade diet.

When feeding commercial pet foods, read the label carefully and always select a high quality combination of ingredients. The total amount of high quality food you'll need to feed each day will definitely be less than the amount of food your pet will require if you're using a lower quality product which is made with a lot of fillers. You'll also find there's usually considerably less stool output when a pet is eating a higher quality food. (*Be sure to refer back to Chapter 1,* **Understanding Commercial Pet Foods**, *for much more information.*)

To determine how much you should feed, you first need to find your pet's ideal weight. You can gauge this fairly well if you can feel his ribs easily when your pet is standing. You shouldn't be able to see them, but if you have to press down to feel the rib bones, or you can't feel them at all, that's a definite sign that there's too much fat. You should also be able to see a noticeable waist below the rib cage.

To monitor your pet's weight more closely, you can weigh him either on a scale at the vet's office, or on a home scale by holding him in your arms, if your pet is small enough, and then subtracting your own weight.

Next, decide what his activity level normally is on a daily basis (couch potato, running circles around the house, jogging every day, etc.).

When you know your pet's ideal weight, you may be able to use one of the charts on the following pages to find a good starting point for how much to feed each day. Remember, though, the approximate weights and quantities of food in each list are only general guidelines.

For dogs (quantity expressed in cups)

Breed Type	Approximate Weight	Dry Food	Moist + Dry Food
Chihuahua, Yorkshire Terrier, Toy Poodle	Up to 10 pounds	1/3 to 1 cup	¼ can + ¾ cup
Miniature Poodle, Bichon Frise, Lahsa Apso, ShihTzu, some Terriers	10 - 25 pounds	1 to 2 ¼ cup	½ can + 1 ½ cup
Cocker Spaniel, Border Collie, Sheep Dogs, Bull Dogs, Hounds, larger Terriers	25 - 50 pounds	2 ¼ to 3 ¼ cups	1 can + 2 ½ cups
Boxer, Collie, Labrador Retriever, Golden Retriever	50 – 75 pounds	3 ¾ to 5 cups	1 ½ can + 3 cups
American Bull Dog, Doberman, Alaskan Malamute, German Shepherd	75 - 100 pounds	5 - 8 cups	2 cans + 5 ¼ cups

For dogs (quantity expressed in ounces)

Breed Type	Approx. Weight	Amount of Food to Feed – in Ounces
Toys: Toy Poodle, Miniature Dachshund, Pekingese, Yorkshire Terrier, etc.	Up to 11 pounds	3 - 5 ounces
Small: Beagle, Jack Russell, Cavalier King Charles, etc	11 - 22 pounds	3.9 - 6.0 ounces
Medium: Basset Hound, Bull Terrier, Springer & Brittany Spaniel, etc.	22 - 55 pounds	10 - 12 ounces
Large: Labrador/Golden Retriever, German Shepherd, Boxer, etc.	55 - 77 pounds	16.0 - 18.2 ounces
Giant: Great Dane, Pyrenees, St. Bernard, etc.	77 pounds and over	24.3 - 30.4 ounces or more

For cats

Age	Body Weight	Ounces of Dry Food	Ounces of Canned Food
10 weeks	2.0 - 2.4 lbs	2.5 - 3.0 oz	7.3 - 8.9 oz
20 weeks	4.2 - 5.5 lbs	2.8 - 3.7 oz	8.0 - 10.5 oz
30 weeks	5.5 - 8.4 lbs	2.8 - 4.2 oz	8.1 - 12.4 oz
40 weeks	6.4 - 8.4 lbs	2.6 - 3.4 oz	7.6 - 9.9 oz
Adult Active	4.8 - 9.9 lbs	2.0 - 4.0 oz	5.7 - 11.8 oz
Adult Inactive	4.8 - 9.9 lbs	1.7 - 3.2 oz	5.0 - 10.3 oz
Senior Adult	4.8 - 9.9 lbs	2.3 - 4.3 oz	6.7 - 7.7 oz
Pregnant	5.5 - 8.0 lbs	2.8 - 4.4 oz	8.1 - 13.0 oz
Nursing	4.8 - 8.8 lbs	6.1 - 11.1 oz	17.8 - 32.4 oz

Feeding pets twice a day is recommended. Once you've decided on the total quantity of food that's right for your pet each day, divide the total amount into two portions. If you're also regularly going to be using treats for training or rewards during the day, you may very likely need to deduct the amount you feed in treats from the total recommended amount you'll be serving at meals.

To be certain you're not overfeeding your pet, you can use either calorie count, if it's provided on the package, or watch how high the protein and fat levels are in each food and treat. If those levels are quite high, you'll either need to decrease the total amount you feed for the day, or select foods and treats with lower levels of protein and fat.

Feed the amount you select for one month and then weigh your pet again. If he's maintaining his ideal weight, you're on the right track. During the month, however, if you discover you can no longer feel your pet's ribs, you may want to check his weight right away and decrease the total amount of food and treats appropriately. And if he seems to be losing too much weight, you may even need to increase the total daily amount of food and treats you feed him.

Adjustments required for different life stages

Puppies and kittens require double the amount of nutrients they'll need when they become adult dogs and cats. These nutrients need to come from food that's specially formulated just for them.

Elderly dogs and cats do need some highly digestible protein every day, but they need less protein than an active adult dog or cat requires.

Giant breed dogs, when growing, should not be free fed or have high calorie diets. Protein levels that are too high may contribute to the development of bone disease in these breeds. The calcium level in their growth diets should also be less than that of a medium or a small breed dog. From 0.8% to 2.00% is acceptable.

A dog who's kept outside during winter should be given up to twice as much protein and fat as an indoor dog.

A nursing mother needs lots of calcium because she can lose about one third of the calcium from her own bones when she's supplying it in her milk. She also needs more food rich in nutrients during pregnancy and when she's nursing.

When and how to feed

There are several effective ways to feed pets. One of the following methods should meet your individual pet's needs. You may even find that you need to use different methods at different stages of your pet's life.

In general, it's best to feed teenage and adult domestic pets twice a day. This enables their bodies to better absorb the nutrients in each serving of food. It may also prevent the kind of gorging on a single meal which can be the cause of painful bloating and gas.

Puppies and kittens, on the other hand, will require multiple feedings throughout the day, but they can benefit from using the Timed Feeding and Portion Control Feeding methods, too.

Timed feeding

This method is recommended for teaching pets to eat when their food is served. It also assures that food isn't left out for long periods of time where it might deteriorate or attract ants, rodents, or other animals, especially if a pet is fed outdoors.

Simply serve food at approximately the same times each day, but leave it down only for 20 minutes. Even if your pet hasn't finished all of it, remove the bowl and dispose of any leftover food. Your pet will quickly learn to satisfy his or her hunger by eating everything that's served before you remove it. Or, after 20 minutes, if there's almost always something leftover, it may mean your pet is actually satisfied with less food than you thought he or she would need.

Portion control feeding

This method is ideal for good weight management, whether a pet is overweight or needs to gain weight gradually. It's a particularly appropriate method for feeding large or giant breed dogs when they're still puppies. If they're allowed to overeat, they may grow too rapidly, which may result in painful bone diseases later on. This method also works well for dogs or cats who would otherwise tend to eat compulsively all day long.

Determine the total amount of food your pet needs each day to maintain good health. Divide this amount into three or four feedings for puppies and kittens, and into two servings for teenage and adult dogs and cats. Serve one portion at each meal.

Remember, if your pet is recovering from surgery or has a medical condition, or if your pet is a nursing mother, you may also need to make other adjustments to meet any special dietary needs.

Free feeding

This method works well for cats, as well as for dogs who don't overeat and aren't overweight. It's also good for nursing mothers. The food you use must not spoil if it's left out for a long time so it's not an appropriate feeding method if you're using a raw food diet or moist canned food. The food also needs to be placed in an area where it won't attract ants, rodents, or other unwelcome critters.

You may leave out any quantity of dry food that will remain fresh for the day, and allow your pet to eat as much or as little as he or she wants. At the end of the day, dispose of any leftover amount and wash the bowl. Don't continually add new food to food that's already been left out for some time.

I personally never like to see food left out all the time because it sometimes creates very finicky eaters. In my experience, animals who have food available all the time tend to have more frequent stomach upsets. Instead of eating in one or two sittings, they munch all day long which can create havoc in their digestive systems because their gastric fluids are constantly working.

An interesting alternative feeding method

One of my editors devised a unique feeding method at a special time in her pet's life. She originally had two Westies who gave each other plenty of exercise, but when the older of the two passed on, she needed to find ways to provide extra fun, exercise and mental stimulation for her then nine-year-old Westie.

Using two different high quality commercial pet foods, she divided the normal morning and evening feeding amounts into approximately six small portions. She served one portion in a bowl, morning and evening, along with moistened nutritional supplements. The remaining four portions were served in her pet's Buster Cube once in the morning and several times during the evening.

By reserving a portion of the total daily amount of food to use in several Buster Cube servings, she could provide the fun, exercise and mental stimulation her pet needed in the absence of a companion, but without the risk of overfeeding, or of any unhealthy weight gain. Peaches is now twelve years old, and her weight remains at a steady and healthy level using this feeding method.

A Buster Cube is a treat dispensing cube which releases pieces of kibble, or other bite-size treats, whenever a pet pushes it quickly around the floor with his or her nose. Most pets travel around and around the room pushing the cube very fast. The fun of finding and eating the pieces of kibble, as they fall out, continually motivates pets to keep working until they can no longer hear the sound of any more kibble rolling around inside. Buster Cubes, and other similar types of treat-dispensing containers, are available in small, medium and large sizes in most pet stores and on internet pet supply web sites.

When you come right down to it, treat dispensing cubes may actually be closer to a more natural way of feeding a pet. Bowls are primarily for our convenience. Animals in the wild don't eat out of bowls. They travel each day, and have to work to find their food, so a treat dispensing toy, filled with a high quality kibble, allows a pet to follow his or her natural hunting instincts and have fun at the same time.

If you'd like to try this method, just be sure to measure out the total amount of food and treats for the whole day first. Then serve divided portions of this total amount in a treat dispensing cube at normal mealtimes, or at any other appropriate times of the day.

Feeding pets who gulp their food

Ideally, you need to be present when your pet is eating, at least until you know how much food he eats at one time, and whether he eats normally or routinely gulps his food down. Knowing how much, and how quickly, your pet eats will enable you to make wise and appropriate modifications to both his diet and his eating behavior.

Gulping food is actually a dangerous activity because, when he gulps food down, a pet also swallows an incredible amount of air at the same time. This combination of food and air in his stomach can cause severe digestive and intestinal problems.

To minimize gulping behavior, you can try placing a large object inside the bowl along with the food. Your pet will then need to take more time, and should ingest smaller bites, as he works his way around the object in order to get at his food.

For instance, try using a ball which is big enough so a pet can't swallow it. You can try using a golf ball for a cat, a baseball for a toy dog, a softball for a medium-size breed, and an even larger ball for large and giant breeds. If your dog is obsessed with balls, then try using an appropriate size polished rock. Whatever object you decide to use, be certain it's smooth and has no sharp edges.

Another technique to reduce the speed with which a dog eats is to scatter dry food over a large area of a floor or patio. When you do this, your pet then has to spend time finding and eating all of the individual pieces of kibble.

Often, in a multiple pet household, gulping behavior is triggered by competition for food, so if you have several pets, it's best to give each pet his or her own bowl rather than using a community feeding bowl.

Water

Every pet needs an ample supply of good clean purified water. Tap water is tempting to use, but it usually contains a number of bacteria as well as harmful chemicals, including chlorine which can cause liver problems. If you can't use bottled water, try to use water from something like a PUR or Britta pitcher with a filter, or a PUR faucet filter which removes chlorine, lead, and bacterial contaminants like giardia.

Since a plentiful quantity of *fresh clean* water should always be available, you may even need to change the water immediately after a pet eats and drinks. Otherwise, the water that's left out may contain food particles or an oily residue from the previous meal.

For pets who are ill, won't eat, or don't want to swallow capsules no matter how cleverly disguised they are, their water can sometimes be used to help them take in some of the nutrients or supplements that would ordinarily be served with their food. For this purpose you might add vitamin/mineral supplements, chlorophyll, apple cider vinegar, aloe vera, or any one of several other beneficial supplements to their water supply. You can find a vitamin supplement especially formulated for this purpose at www.pawier.com.

If you need to use water to help provide supplementation, there are a couple of precautions you'll need to take. To be sure your pet receives an adequate amount of the supplement, put whatever you're adding into only a minimal amount of water and be sure he or she consumes as much of that water solution as possible. Also have additional fresh water ready for use as soon as the treated supply is finished.

Pets who are sick may not like the taste of water with something added to it, so you may also need to offer plain water in between times to be sure they remain as well hydrated as possible.

Food and water containers

The best containers to use are those made of stainless steel, glass or ceramic. If you're using a glass or ceramic bowl, be very certain it's lead-free. If you can't be certain, then choose a different type of bowl.

Why be so cautious about the bowl you use, and why aren't plastic bowls recommended? Water is like a solvent. It tends to dissolve materials in a container and absorb them into itself. Some foods tend to do the same thing.

Pet and other specialty stores have an abundant supply of plastic containers for both dogs and cats. Most are made of materials recognized as "food grade" plastic. But knowing that your pet's food or water could be absorbing chemicals from the plastic in their bowls, wouldn't you want to avoid creating a potentially toxic hazard for them?

Monitoring changes in diet

Whenever you're making changes in your pet's diet, you need to be aware of what effects those changes may be having, positive or not so positive. Here are several guidelines to help keep any negative effects to a minimum:

- Introduce only one new food item, supplement or treat at a time.
- Introduce new foods gradually, and only in small quantities at a time.
- Mentally, or in writing, keep track of all of the different foods, supplements or treats your pet is eating so you can review what you've most recently added. It may even take a day or more before you see any changes resulting from the addition of something new.
- Keep an eye on how foods, supplements and treats affect your dog or cat by checking their stools regularly. Are they very soft and loose, rather than formed and of normal consistency? If so, there are several possible reasons. Chances are, changes in the diet are being made too quickly, the food is not being digested properly, or the food is lacking in the necessary enzymes to facilitate digestion.
- If a pet has excessive gas, the fruits and vegetables you're using may be of the gas forming variety and need to be eliminated, or the quantity may simply need to be reduced. Be sure to change or add only one new item at a time so you'll know exactly which food is causing any problem.

The fine art of poop watching

Poop watching is a way of practicing good preventive medicine.

In the days of courts and jesters, the royal doctor cared for the well being of the royal family. Part of his responsibility was to inspect, in detail, everything that came out of the bodies of each of the royal family members. This meant he needed to actually look at their urine and bowel movements to determine, just by observation, if there was any cause for medical concern.

We also need to be like royal doctors for our pets. You may not regard poop watching as one of your favorite activities, but whenever you do have pets, it needs to be one of your daily responsibilities.

Poop watching serves two purposes:

1. It helps you be aware of whether your pets are in good health or if they may need medical attention.
2. You'll be able to see if your animals are eating things that are unusual, things they're not supposed to eat, or if they're getting into anything that could be harmful to their well-being.

Here's what you need to look for:

- Good excrement should be firm, dark brown, well-shaped and compact.
- Soft or runny stools can alert you to the need for a change in diet, or the presence of possible illness.
- Slimy stools, or stools coated with mucus, may be an indication that there's not enough fiber in the diet, or they may be a sign of constipation or other digestive problems.
- Copious amounts of stool may mean that not enough food is actually being digested and metabolized.
- More than two stools per day may be an indication of overfeeding.
- Look for worms or white specks *immediately* after a pet has an elimination. If the stool has been on the ground for any length of time before you see it, be sure the white specks aren't something coming up off the grass or from the soil.
- Look for blood, or for dark spots which may indicate the presence of blood.
- Look for stringy pieces of grass, yarn, household objects, twigs, candy wrappers or un-digested pieces of food like carrots.

Whenever you're in doubt, take a sample to your veterinarian and have it analyzed.

Other poopy problems

Partially evacuated objects

On rare occasions, you may discover that a pet hasn't been able to completely evacuate part of a stool that contains an unusual object like a foil candy wrapper or yarn. In this case, if you think you can safely remove the object because it's already almost fully out, *do so very slowly and carefully*. Usually, though, it's best to leave the object in place exactly as it is and let your veterinarian remove it. You may not know how much of it is still traveling through the intestine in the case of yarn, or it may be sharp enough to cut the intestinal wall or rectum, as in the case of foil wrappers.

Copraphagia

You may also observe your pet eating his own excrement, or that of other dogs or cats. This is called copraphagia. We humans consider this a very unsavory habit, but animals have several reasons for doing it. They may be searching for something that's missing in their diets, the excrement they find may contain a lot of tasty (to them) undigested protein (this is especially true of cat poop), or they may simply consider eating poop a fun thing to do.

This kind of behavior may, in some cases, even represent a natural way of meeting dietary needs. For dogs in the wild, eating soil is a way of obtaining minerals, while eating bark from trees provides an important source of fiber for them. They even find some valuable nutrients in material that we humans find totally repugnant, like vomit, decaying flesh, and feces. Feces, for them, may even be a highly valuable food if it contains quantities of good bacteria.

Although eating feces is usually considered a behavioral problem in domesticated animals, we're now learning that this type of behavior might be caused by a nutritional deficiency. If there aren't sufficient nutrients in a pet's food to provide all of the nutrition he needs, then he won't be able to maintain a steady weight, and may remain hungry much of the time. This may cause him to search for those nutrients in undesirable ways. Usually, dogs fed a well-balanced natural diet or a high quality commercial pet food diet are less likely to eat their own feces than dogs who eat a lower grade commercial pet food diet.

If you add supplements to a pet's regular food, like kelp or pet formulated minerals, the temptation to eat poop may be considerably minimized. Also consider adding other nutritious ingredients like yogurt, eggs, oils containing essential fatty acids, enzyme supplements, antioxidants, and fiber.

* * *

In the next chapter, we'll look at foods which all pets should avoid or which should be used only with caution.

Chapter 6

Foods All Pets Should Avoid

Although it seems that some pets are able to eat almost anything without any unpleasant consequences, there are still some basic food guidelines we should follow for all pets.

Foods to avoid — general guidelines

The following foods should not be fed to pets, either because they're not healthy for them, or because they may not be compatible with a pet's digestive system:

- No bacon, bacon grease, or other leftover fats (as much as they may like them!)
- No ham or other pork products (ham is too salty)
- No spicy foods (chili, pepperoni, hot peppers or other highly seasoned foods)
- No fried foods, sauces or very salty foods
- No cookies, cakes, ice cream, candy or other sweets
- No sugarless candies or gum containing Xylitol
- No chocolate (chocolate in most forms can be toxic and even deadly)
- No cheeses (cheese is too fattening to be used for regular feeding, though it can be used as a very effective training treat in limited quantities)

As a general rule, never give cat food to dogs and never give dog food to cats.

Cat food is too high in protein and fat for dogs, and dog food doesn't have the right balance of nutrients for cats. Long-term feeding of dog food to cats may cause malnutrition.

For cats, canned tuna intended for human consumption is not recommended on a regular basis (more than once a week). This type of canned tuna often has a higher mercury content than cat food tuna does. If you're using human canned tuna as a treat, use the kind packed in water.

The oil in regular canned tuna, used over a long period of time, can deplete vitamin E, possibly resulting in fatty liver disease (steatites). Canned tuna for people doesn't provide the necessary balance of nutrients for cats, so prolonged feeding could result in malnutrition unless supplemented with vitamin E, taurine and veggies.

Specific foods that should be avoided or used only with caution for dogs and cats

It's not wise to assume that human foods are also good for pets. The following list provides additional information about many of those foods and why they should be avoided altogether, or at least used with caution.

- **Alcoholic Beverages**—may cause coma and death from intoxication.
- **Avocado**—the leaves and bark of the avocado tree, and the seeds and skin of the fruit are toxic to pets and can affect the heart; the fruit itself, however, has nutritional benefits.
- **Baby Food**—may contain onion powder which can be toxic for dogs and cats. Baby Food is also not nutritionally balanced for dogs or cats for long term feeding. However, using certain baby foods can be a godsend when you need to feed a pureed diet to a sick or injured pet, or one who is recovering from surgery. Just be sure the food you choose doesn't contain onions, onion powder, or onion salt.
- **Bones**—cooked bones can splinter and cause obstructions or lacerations. Raw bones should not pose this problem. Bones are not appropriate for pets who don't have strong healthy teeth.
- **Broccoli**—best fed in small quantities; if broccoli is steamed this may remove the element that is considered potentially toxic but hasn't yet been proven to cause health threats; broccoli can be fed at less than 10% of the diet since it's rich in vitamins and minerals and is good for the immune system with its antioxidant and anti-cancerous properties.
- **Chewing Gum**—sugar-free chewing gum contains Xylitol, which may cause too much insulin to be released. Symptoms may start within 30 minutes and last for several hours. You should have your pet evaluated by a veterinarian for treatment.
- **Chocolate**—contains theobromine; semi-sweet and bakers chocolate contain significantly higher amounts than milk

chocolate; cocoa powder and cooking chocolate are very toxic; pets may experience anything from digestive problems to death; activated charcoal may keep a pet from absorbing too much; there's no specific antidote; signs of toxicity may not show up immediately; contact your vet right away.

- **Coffee, Tea and Caffeine**—caffeine can be toxic and fatal at 150mg/kg of body weight; there's no antidote; contact your vet immediately.
- **Citrus Oil Extracts**—may cause vomiting.
- **Eggs** (raw)—may decrease the absorption of the B vitamin Biotin which could cause skin and hair coat problems; the Biotin deficiency may be avoided by cooking the eggs or feeding only the raw yolk and not the raw white; raw eggs are thought to be a source of salmonella, though this may be more true for ordinary store bought eggs than for organic free range eggs according to those who frequently eat raw eggs.
- **Fat Trimmings**—may cause pancreatitis.
- **Fish** (raw)—if fed regularly, raw fish may cause a deficiency of the B vitamin thiamin which may result in loss of appetite and seizures, or in severe cases, death; raw salmon may cause salmon poisoning disease with the symptoms resembling those of canine parvovirus.
- **Garlic**—contains some elements which, if fed in large enough quantities, can damage red blood cells causing anemia; is often used in small amounts to treat allergies, infections and as a flea preventative; is less toxic than onions which contain the same elements.
- **Grapes and Raisins**—may cause kidney failure because of a currently unidentified toxin; seek veterinary help right away; the recommendation is to avoid grapes and raisins altogether.
- **Hops**—may lead to seizures and death.
- **Iron**—may be toxic to the liver and kidneys; may damage the lining of the digestive system; found in many vitamins for humans.
- **Liver**—too much may cause vitamin A toxicity which affects muscles and bones.
- **Macadamia Nuts**—contain an unidentified toxin which may be harmful to the nervous system, digestive system and muscles.

- **Marijuana**—may affect the heart rate, depress the nervous system, and cause vomiting.
- **Milk and Dairy Products**—contain lactose; may cause diarrhea; many pets lack the digestive enzyme lactase which breaks down lactose; look for lactose free products specifically made for pets.
- **Moldy or Spoiled Food or Garbage**—may cause vomiting and diarrhea because it contains multiple toxins; severe reactions may affect bodily organs.
- **Mushrooms**—*some* varieties are highly toxic; though most backyard mushrooms are not in this category it's still wise to dig them up completely right away, especially if you have a curious puppy or kitten; toxic varieties may cause coma or death; less toxic varieties may cause diarrhea, reduced pulse rate, disorientation and excess salivation; best to seek veterinary attention immediately.
- **Onions**—contain elements which can be highly toxic to pets if ingested in large quantities or fed repeatedly in small quantities; can cause red blood cells to burst; without red blood cells to carry oxygen, pets can become short of breath; pets may become anemic; avoid baby foods, broths, sauces, and table scraps, pizza, Chinese food, etc. which may contain onions; also avoid raw, cooked, whole, chopped, dehydrated and powdered onions; be aware that onions may be part of seasonings and broths even if they're not specifically listed on the label.
- **Persimmons**—seeds may cause inflammation, or an obstruction in the intestines.
- **Pits from Fruits**—may cause obstructions in the digestive tract; some pits—such as plums, peaches and apricots—may also contain an element which can lead to cyanide poisoning; the same is true for the cores and seeds of pears and apples.
- **Potatoes**—peelings, stems, sprouted parts and green looking potatoes contain oxylates which may affect a pet's digestive, nervous and urinary tract systems.
- **Rhubarb**—leaves contain oxalates which may affect the digestive, nervous and urinary tract systems.
- **Salt**—consuming too much may lead to electrolyte (sodium, potassium, chloride) imbalances; sources include ice melts, rock

salt, and regular salt; salt ingestion may be treatable, though dogs have succumbed after consuming large quantities.

- **String**—may become trapped in the digestive system; pet may show signs of gastrointestinal distress; if an end of the string appears to be coming out of the anus, don't pull on it; seek veterinary help immediately.
- **Sugar and Sugary Foods**—may lead to dehydration or bacterial overload or imbalance in the digestive system; also may lead to obesity, diabetes, and dental problems.
- **Table scraps**—never feed in large amounts; make table scraps *less* than 10% of a pet's diet; they aren't nutritionally balanced; they may contain large quantities of onions, garlic and mushrooms; they may include excessive fat, unless it's been trimmed away from the meat.
- **Tobacco**—nicotine in tobacco products may cause rapid heart beat, collapse, coma and even death.
- **Tomato**—leaves and stems contain oxylates which may affect a pet's digestive, nervous and urinary tract systems.
- **Xylitol**—an ingredient in sugarless candies and chewing gum; has been determined by the National Animal Poison Control Center to be a risk to pets; may cause liver damage.
- **Yeast Dough**—may expand producing excessive gas in the digestive system; this may cause pain or even possible rupture of the stomach or intestines.

For a wealth of additional information on the Internet, do a search on (item name) for dogs (such as chocolate for dogs, or chocolate toxicity for dogs), or (item name) for cats. You can also use (item name)+dogs, or (item name)+cats.

* * *

In the next three chapters, I'll provide information that can be used for pets who are facing some of the most difficult health challenges, plus a number of recipes for those who have special dietary needs.

Chapter 7

Nutritional Support
For Major Health Challenges

Nowadays, our pets' diets often need to be designed to meet a variety of very unique health challenges. These may include major diseases, recovery from surgery, chronic diseases and conditions, allergies, skin problems, weight management and aging.

While doing research for this book, I came across a wealth of information about these topics, and I'm including as much of that information as possible in the next several chapters for those readers who are searching for this type of guidance.

In this chapter we'll look at some of the bigger health challenges our pets face and how we can use good nutrition to support them. We'll also talk about the role fasting plays in the healing process.

Cancer

The diet for a pet with cancer needs to be higher in protein, complex carbohydrates and essential fatty acids, and lower in simple carbohydrates. The increased protein and good fats are required to meet the body's increased energy demands during illness. Protein provides the building blocks to repair cells, tissues and organs. Essential fatty acids, especially omega-3s, help the body fight infection, strengthen the immune system, and repair cell membranes.

Some of the foods best known for fighting cancer are fresh, raw, organically grown vegetables and fruits. Fresh carrot juice, or carrot juice combined with beet and celery juice, provides some excellent sources of nutrients. The same is true for fresh juices made with grapes and apples. Although the skins and seeds of grapes are among the foods for pets to avoid, the juice from the fruit itself should not cause a problem.

Lactic acid generating vegetables, like natural pickles made without vinegar, are excellent for improving digestion. They may also help prevent the nausea sometimes associated with chemotherapy.

Good herbal additions for pets with cancer include garlic, ginger, sage, thyme, eucalyptus, wormwood and rue. Supplements such as apple cider vinegar, garlic vinegar, yogurt, kefir, acidophilus and digestive enzymes may also help.

Diabetes

Keys to a good diabetic diet include limiting simple carbohydrates and maintaining a good balance of protein, fat, complex carbohydrates and fiber. Simple carbohydrates include sucrose (table sugar), lactose (milk sugar), and fructose (the sugar found in fruits, veggies and high fructose corn syrup). Fruits should be used in moderation in pets with diabetes because they are a source of fructose. Fiber helps the body absorb carbohydrates more slowly, and this helps to keep blood sugar levels more stable. Higher levels of l-Carnitine are also necessary to help the body utilize fat more effectively.

Heart disease

Heart disease in dogs can range from mild to serious. Some of the causes include genetic defects, heartworm infestation, inadequate nutrition, and diseases which affect the heart muscle.

Your veterinarian will probably describe a pet's level of heart disease as being Stage 1, 2, 3 or 4. How you'll use good nutrition to treat heart disease depends on what stage your pet's condition has progressed to when the diagnosis is made. Dietary restrictions usually only become necessary if a pet is retaining fluid, has high blood pressure, or is taking certain medications.

Protein is very important for dogs with heart disease. During the later stages, it may need to be reduced somewhat, but it should never be restricted in the early stages of heart disease because this can put more stress on the heart and cause it to lose muscle mass. Use a high quality animal protein, either raw or lightly cooked. Avoid high-temperature cooking because it can destroy taurine, which is necessary for heart health in dogs. Feeding red meats is helpful because they contain l-Carnitine which also helps to support the cells of the heart muscle.

Sodium or salt restriction is not usually necessary in the first stages of heart disease, but it does become important in Stages 3 and 4. Most raw diets, or home cooked diets, are fine for dogs with heart disease because they're naturally low in sodium. Fresh foods, including meat, eggs, vegetables and dairy (except cottage cheese, which is high in sodium) can be used. Don't feed ham, bacon or other smoked meats, however, because these are very high in sodium. Low quality commercial pet foods are also often high in sodium when it's used as a preservative.

When a dog has heart disease, it's important to maintain a normal healthy weight to avoid putting extra stress on the heart. Fats in the diet should be used in moderation. If a dog is overweight, or in class 3 or 4 heart failure, be sure to trim or drain excess fat, avoid high fat foods (lamb, goat, pork) and remove skin from all poultry.

Supplements that have been identified as supporting heart function for our pets include fish or salmon oils, and vitamins E, B-Complex, and C. Other helpful supplements include Taurine, l-Carnitine and CoQ10.

Pets with heart disease must often be treated with a number of medications, including diuretics. Since diuretics tend to quickly deplete the body of many nutrients before they've even been absorbed, it's important to provide high enough levels of vitamins and minerals to compensate for this loss. It's also important to check with your vet about the supplements you want to give your pet to be sure they won't interfere with, or be affected by, any medications your pet is taking.

Liver disease

The liver may be the most important cleansing organ in the body because it must process *everything* the body takes in. This includes not only the good food your pet eats, but also substances such as food preservatives and colorings, antibiotics, medications, insecticides, air pollution, chemicals from household cleaners and aerosol sprays, and excess hormones such as insulin. The liver also has to process all of the fat and junk food your pet eats.

As I've been writing this chapter, I've been helping a client family who just lost their pet to liver disease because it wasn't diagnosed early enough. Their pet's story helps to illustrate some of the warning symptoms of liver disease.

Tramp was a wonderful animal soul who was adopted from the shelter as an adult dog and lived with his new family for almost nine years. He was quite a character, and his outlook on life was always positive and full of enthusiasm.

Tramp started developing sores on his paws. He'd lick them until they became red and were almost infected. The veterinarian thought this might be an irritation caused by an allergy. Tramp was then treated accordingly, including a change in diet. But no amount of dietary changes, antihistamines, creams, soaks, supplements, herbs such as milk thistle, shots, or medications were working.

When he came to see me recently, I saw scabs on all four of his paws from sores that weren't healing. I knew something was very wrong. The family decided to consult another veterinarian who recognized right away that the toxins in his body were not being processed because Tramp was already in the final stages of liver disease.

The skin has sometimes been called a secondary liver because, when the liver isn't able to process everything in a timely manner, some of the toxins may try to exit the body through the skin. A skin breakdown in the feet that won't heal and quickly spreads to the legs is a classic indication of impaired liver function. Other signs may include sores around the mouth, which Tramp also had. All of these symptoms were beginning to show up because his liver wasn't able to do its job properly, and Tramp finally lost his battle to live on Januray 29, 2007. Had he been correctly diagnosed earlier, however, there are many dietary recommendations and nutritional supplements which might have helped him enjoy a longer life.

One of my editors also had a pet with liver disease who manifested some entirely different symptoms and behaviors.

Casey ate a high quality diet, received veterinarian approved nutritional supplements plus vitamins and minerals, and drank purified water all of his life. Yet, in the last several years before his condition was finally diagnosed, his stools were never really well formed and of normal consistency; he occasionally tended to spit up some yellowish fluid the first thing in the morning before he'd eaten anything; and once in awhile, he threw up what he *had* eaten. He was also forever trying to eat anything he could find on his daily walks, especially poop, either his own, or that of other dogs and cats.

He still enjoyed his walks, but began to walk much more slowly than Peaches, his friend and companion, who was only a year younger. At first his mom attributed this to the fact that he was, after all, getting older. But when he went into his bed at night, he just seemed to plop down and look up at her as if to say, "Well, I made it through another day, but I'm just so exhausted."

Excessive barking was another problem that began in the later stages of the disease before she even knew that his liver had begun to fail. This probably happened because he wasn't feeling physically well any longer, and it was more difficult for him to tolerate anything that altered his ordinary routine.

All of these symptoms and behaviors went on for several years, and were regularly brought to the attention of competent veterinarians, but regular visits to the vet and repeated laboratory tests never showed the expected signs of any physical abnormality, including serious liver problems. Constant attention to what he was eating, and using different supplements, didn't produce any positive changes either.

With 20/20 hindsight, she says that if she ever observed these behaviors in another one of her pets, the first thing she would think about, even in the presence of normal laboratory tests, would be intense nutritional support specifically designed for the liver.

Two products, recommended to her by holistic veterinarians, include Natural Factors Milk Thistle Phytosome (www.naturalfactors.com) and Himalaya Herbal Health Care's Liv.52 Vet (www.himalayahealthcare.com). The Milk Thistle Phytosome complex includes 150 mg of milk thistle, plus dandelion, artichoke and turmeric, while the Liv.52 Vet formula contains herbs which have successfully been used by Tibetan doctors for thousands of years.

Since standard laboratory tests may not show early evidence of liver problems, she'd also ask her veterinarian to perform a bile acid response test in the presence of symptoms and behaviors like those listed above.

This test is started after at least a twelve hour fast by drawing a sample of blood to obtain a baseline value for bile acids. A small meal is fed right away, and then blood is drawn again in two hours. If the bile acids are elevated significantly on either test, or if there is a significant rise in bile acids between the first and second blood samples, then it's likely there's a decrease in the functional capacity of the liver.

While an overburdened liver may become seriously diseased, if treatment is started in time, the liver has an almost miraculous ability to completely recover when it's provided with the proper nutrients. High quality protein, highly digestible complex carbohydrates, specific vitamins and minerals, milk thistle and dandelion supplements, and reducing the amount of toxins that have to be processed can all help the liver regenerate itself.

Even after finally being diagnosed with full blown end-stage liver disease, Casey still continued to enjoy life as much as he could for another six months until it was finally time for him to cross over The Rainbow Bridge. You can read his full story in the last chapter of my second book *Pets Have Feelings Too!*

If you notice any of the same symptoms or behaviors in your own pets that either Tramp or Casey exhibited, you might want to consider starting a high level of liver support, and ask for specialized testing.

Kidney disease

Kidney failure is the inability of the kidneys to remove waste products from the blood. It is *not* the inability to create urine. Ironically, most pets with kidney failure are actually producing large quantities of urine, but kidney function has deteriorated to the point that waste products from the body are not being properly eliminated.

The responsibility of the kidneys is to filter poisons, wastes and foreign chemicals out of the blood so that they can be eliminated normally by the body. Often, the kidneys have had to process an excess amount of amino acids from the poor quality protein found in many commercial pet foods, or from a diet that consists mainly of protein. When this happens over an extended period of time, the kidneys may stop functioning properly.

Lower salt intake and essential fatty acids can help slow the progression of kidney disease. It's important for a pet with kidney problems to consume plenty of water to keep the urine output well diluted and flowing freely.

If your pet does have kidney disease, it's also important to reduce the amount of protein and phosphorus in the diet, and provide higher amounts of fiber and complex carbohydrates. Some veterinarians also suggest using a low ash diet for pets with kidney disease. This requires avoiding the use of organ meats and high ash foods such as dry foods and fish.

A low ash diet, however, may have to be used with some caution. Why?

Ash is the inorganic residue that's left after heating the food to around 550 degrees Celsius. It comes from bones and is part of the "meal." The higher the ash content of a food, the higher the mineral content will be. Ash includes all of the minerals necessary to support normal bodily functions. It supplies calcium, magnesium, phosphorus, and other trace minerals. Consequently, in a low ash diet, there may be insufficient amounts of these minerals to keep a pet healthy.

Some studies have shown that magnesium is so important for bodily functions that if the body is depleted of this important mineral, then the original problem may be intensified instead of being corrected. If your pet does need to be on a low ash diet, it may therefore be important to give magnesium and other minerals in supplemental form.

Talk with your veterinarian and do your own research before deciding whether or not your pet with kidney disease will benefit from a low ash diet. Too much ash in a pet's diet may set the stage for kidney stones and bladder infections, but too little ash may deprive your pet of some important nutrients. You need to find the right balance for your own pet.

Urinary tract problems

Urinary tract problems include infections, inflammation (cystitis), and kidney or bladder stones. Symptoms you can look for include going frequently but producing only small amounts of urine each time, blood in the urine, obvious pain when urinating, and straining or being reluctant to go because of the discomfort.

It's not unusual to have microscopic-size mineral crystals in the urine, and these very small crystals usually pass normally. But when these crystals tend to clump together forming stones, they may cause major problems. Sometimes your pet may not show any symptoms when this happens, but a veterinarian may be able to feel some of the larger stones when he presses on the bladder during an examination. X-rays and ultrasound can also be used to locate stones.

There are many reasons why pets develop kidney stones. A high protein diet in itself may be a contributing factor, but while the amount of protein may contribute to the problem, the type and/or quality of protein may be even more important. High purine-yielding foods like liver and organ meats definitely need to be avoided. Pets who don't drink enough water or who don't have the opportunity to empty their bladders when they need to may also be more likely to develop stones. And then there are certain breeds who seem to be more genetically predisposed to kidney and bladder problems than others.

Stones usually develop in the kidneys and/or bladder. Kidney stones may then be found in the ureters when they're trying to pass on through. (The ureters are long narrow tubes which connect the kidneys to the bladder.) And both kidney and bladder stones may be found in the urethra, the small tube through which urine passes to the outside. The ureters and urethra are all narrow tubes so that the accumulation of any sizeable crystals in them has the potential to cause an obstruction and prevent the passage of urine. The urethras in male dogs and cats are narrower than those in female dogs and cats, so males may experience complete urethral blockages more than females do.

Kidney stones are made of calcified material. Fortunately, they occur far less often in dogs and cats than bladder stones, but the possibility of kidney stones should always be considered in urinary tract disease. These stones may cause sudden colic and intermittent bloody urine or may occur without any visible symptoms. Many times pets live with kidney stones for years without noticeable ill effects.

Bladder stones, on the other hand, are mineral formations that come about when the urine becomes too alkaline. An alkaline environment also seems to cause bacteria to grow faster. If a bacterial infection does occur, the waste products from those bacteria further increase the unhealthy alkaline environment of the bladder. The bacteria may even provide a solid object to which dissolved minerals can attach, but keeping the urine acidic helps to prevent these problems from developing. In dogs and cats, grain-based diets contribute to alkaline urine, while meat-based diets promote the more desirable acidic urine.

Stones are usually identified in one of three ways: struvite, oxalate and urate.

Struvite crystals are more common in females and may be encouraged to dissolve with a reduced protein diet which reduces the amount of ammonia formed in the urine. When they're present in the bladder in small amounts, these crystals usually pass normally, but if they're present in large amounts, they tend to form stones.

Urate stones are composed of one or more types of purines but they may also be dissolved with a diet which is low in purines, though your pet may also require anti-purine medications in addition to dietary changes.

Oxalate stones, which can form even in acidic urine, are more often found in males. They're less likely to respond to diet and medications and usually need to be removed surgically. They result from too much calcium in the blood and urine, excessive use of cortecosteroids or Cushing's disease. Dietary changes don't usually have any positive effect on oxalate stones.

If you have a cat who's suddenly "missing" the litterbox and urinating in other places around the house, it would be very wise to check for a bladder infection or stones. Pain or discomfort in the cat's bladder when it urinates is sometimes perceived by the cat as the fault of the litterbox! Because the cat thinks the litterbox is causing the pain, he or she seeks out a safer and more comfortable area in which to eliminate, such as the owner's bed, a laundry basket, on or behind couches, in a tub or sink, or in closets and other dark corners.

My experience with my own Shih-Tzu, Chop Chop, taught me that a pet can have all three types of stones at the same time, and that they can be located in multiple places all at the same time. This can be a life-threatening situation, especially for a pet who is older or not in good health. Multiple surgeries are usually the only option at this point if a pet is even able to tolerate such intense surgeries. Without quick medical intervention (within hours or a very few days), an animal will die from major obstructions caused by kidney or bladder stones because the body is no longer able to rid itself of toxins.

As you can see, some urinary tract problems can be painful and even fatal if they're not discovered and treated in time. But there's good news, too.

Infections, inflammation and stones can be treated in several different ways. Dietary changes, increased water intake, and medications, including antibiotics, may be sufficient if there's no blockage. However if a blockage occurs, immediate surgery may be required.

Reducing the levels of protein and phosphorus in the diet helps to keep the urine more acidic. This in turn will help reduce the formation of crystals which may otherwise eventually group together to form stones. However, dogs should not be left on a reduced protein diet for more than five or six months, though cats may be able to follow the restricted diet for a little longer.

Other ways to make the urine more acidic include using appropriate amounts of vitamin C and cranberry juice, or cranberry in capsule form. Cranberry capsules may be the better form since cranberry juice contains such high amounts of simple sugar.

Other helpful supplements to use when your pet has urinary tract problems include vitamins A and B, especially B6 which acts like a diuretic. B vitamins can be obtained from a B-Complex supplement or from brewer's yeast.

Another suggestion is to make a tea from the roots of couch or quack grasses by boiling 1 ½ cups of water, bruising the root, and letting it simmer for four hours. Before meals, give 1-4 tablespoons to your dog, or one tablespoon to your cat.

You'll also need to encourage your pets with urinary tract problems to drink plenty of water. If you need to entice them to drink more water, add a tiny pinch of salt to their food. This will make them thirsty enough to drink more, which will both dilute and increase the overall amount of urine.

Gastrointestinal disorders and diarrhea

Animals who scavange, or eat almost anything, are the ones most likely to suffer from gastrointestinal problems, and some pets, especially those with Irritable Bowel Syndrome, may have frequent diarrhea. Some animals will instinctively try to remedy gastrointestinal discomfort by eating grass which induces vomiting. At the first sign of any type of upset, provide your pet with plenty of fresh water or ice cubes to lick, but have him fast from all food for 24 hours.

When you re-introduce food again, start with a bland diet of rice, then gradually add a little cottage cheese and additional protein in the form of boiled skinless chicken breast. Feed small meals several times a day, and massage the stomach area to stimulate motion in the intestines.

Although there can be many causes of gastrointestinal upsets, one factor that comes up over and over again is an intolerance for grains in the diet, especially wheat. You'll need to check the ingredients in both the food and the treats your pet is eating because wheat is often a primary ingredient.

Many dogs who are switched to a grain-free raw diet, including raw meaty bones and pureed veggies, do very well, often better than they have in their entire lives. A grain-free cooked diet also works well. In general, for a pet with frequent gastrointestinal distress, stay away from all grains and other starchy foods that take a long time to digest (like potatoes and corn), limit the amount of fiber (from vegetables), and avoid dairy.

Some studies have been done that indicate supplementing with omega-3 fatty acids like fish oil can help with intestinal inflammation. One recommendation suggests giving a maximum of 1 gram (1000 mg) per 10 pounds of bodyweight. This amount should generally include 300 mg of DHA and EPA fatty acids. Be sure to also give vitamin E whenever you supplement with oils.

Irritable bowel syndrome

If a pet with Irritable Bowel Syndrome is having diarrhea, follow the guidelines in the section above first. Also stop using all treats and edible chews during an outbreak, no matter how much your pet begs.

Once the diarrhea is under control, the first step in managing Irritable Bowel Syndrome on a long term basis is fat restriction because fat prolongs the amount of time food spends in the stomach. The second step is to introduce a different type of diet which is unfamiliar to the animal's body. Proteins like rabbit, venison or duck are typically used when making this kind of a change. Some fresh lamb might also be appropriate if your pet hasn't ever eaten it before.

Although home cooking used to be the only option when a pet required allergen free meals, there are now some high quality commercial pet foods which use alternative proteins and good carbohydrates without the use of additives. Some of the new menu choices include venison and potato, fish and potato, egg and rice, duck and peas (excellent for cats) and even kangaroo meat.

If you're using a homemade diet, be sure to use only soluble fibers. Although you may think of them as starch, they can't be digested by enzymes in the gastrointestinal track and are therefore passed quickly through the body.

Examples of soluble fibers are:

Rice	Carrots	Beets	Papayas *(also*
Rice Cereals	Yams	Squash	*act as a diges-*
Oatmeal	Sweet	Pumpkin	*tive aid to*
Barley	potatoes	Chestnuts	*relieve gas and*
Quinoa	Turnips	Bananas	*indigestion)*
Corn meal	Rutabagas	Applesauce	
Potatoes	Parsnips	Mangoes*	

** Fruit only; mango skins may cause mouth irritation*

Continue using a diet of natural whole foods consisting of highly digestible proteins, complex carbohydrates, good fats, and additional fiber, along with probiotics which are very beneficial for proper intestinal function. Remember the main diet: 60-80 % protein, with the other 20-40% divided about equally between complex carbohydrates and raw vegetables.

Add some Slippery Elm Bark and you should have a handle on the problem.

Recovery from surgery or illnesses

This type of diet should be high in protein and essential fatty acids (the good fats) to help prevent loss of lean body mass and maintain body defenses. In general, also add amino acids, vitamins, omega-3 fatty acids and minerals. A semi-liquid or soft diet may be beneficial to use for awhile for animals who are recuperating from surgery. Some people find it helpful to puree whole organic foods or to use pureed baby foods during their pet's recovery period, but be sure to avoid baby foods with any added salt, onions, onion salt or onion powder.

The importance of fasting

We worry when our pets stop eating and we often try to entice them to eat by adding gravy or tasty morsels to their food, but this isn't necessary. Some pets may go a whole day without eating and then eat very normally the next day.

Instinctively, animals know when fasting will help their bodies recover from whatever is causing them discomfort. They may approach their food bowl but turn around immediately and walk away, or stare at the food and then at you. This is normal, and at times like these, you shouldn't make your pets eat or tempt them with treats that may only make them feel worse. Think of how you feel when you're sick with a cold or the flu. You're not that hungry, and you'd rather just sleep than eat a meal.

Instead, try to offer your pet some unsalted or low-sodium broth (chicken or vegetable) to provide some nourishment. Usually a pet fasts for only one day, and by the next morning he or she is hungry again, if not downright ravenous. If a pet doesn't eat for three days, then it's time to consult your veterinarian. If a pet stops drinking water for more than one day, consult your veterinarian right away.

In the past, I've had clients who have fasted their pets one day a week on purpose because it benefited their pets' overall health. And in the wild, animals will fast one out of every seven to ten days.

Fasting an animal when he or she is sick is not only beneficial but sometimes even necessary. It gives the body a chance to detoxify and clear out substances that are causing discomfort, or are otherwise detrimental. During the time pets are fasting, they can use all of their energy to fight any germs, viruses or parasites.

Fasting for a day is also a great way to entice super finicky animals to eat. This means you shouldn't offer them any food or treats for a whole day, but instead provide plenty of water, love and games. The next day, when you feed them the same food they were finicky about before, the scent may now trigger a thought that says, "Yummy, I'm hungry! Let's eat!"

Another way to help a finicky dog want to eat is to make him hungry by taking him for an energetic walk (not the stop, smell, and pee kind), but a fast walk for exercise purposes. You'll soon see that, upon returning home, your pet will go straight to the bowl, quite content to eat the whole meal.

* * *

Absolutely everything begins with good nutrition, especially when our pets are facing health challenges of any kind, so a high level of nutrition is always the first step you need to take on the road to healing or maintaining optimum health.

In the next two chapters, you'll find a wide variety of helpful recipes you can use whenever your pet is experiencing some type of health challenge or has a special dietary need.

Chapter 8

Recipes Designed For Pets With Major Health Challenges

The following recipes are each designed for small breed dogs weighing up to about 20 pounds. Consequently, the quantities in each recipe will need to be significantly increased for larger dogs, or the serving sizes will need to be decreased for very small dogs.

The total number of meals you'll be able to serve from a single recipe will depend on how much food your pet needs to eat in a day. This usually depends on an individual pet's weight and appetite. Feed two servings each day unless otherwise indicated in the recipe.

As a rule of thumb, it's always wise to feed animals twice a day. However, when animals are ill, they aren't always able to consume a full size serving at a single meal. When this happens, it's better to divide the total amount of food into four separate feedings per day to be sure your pet is eating enough to receive all of the nutrients she needs.

If you're preparing home made food for your pet, when should you add the vitamins, minerals and other nutritional supplements?

Whenever you're adding vitamins, minerals and other nutritional supplements to home made meals, always add them *after* all of the other ingredients have been blended together and cooled somewhat. Then mix them in gently *by hand*.

Can nutritional supplements be added all at one time to the total day's food supply?

This means you'd be making up a quantity of food sufficient for one day and mixing all of the supplements for that day into the large batch. The total amount of food, with supplements already in it, would then be divided into two or more servings. Some professionals say yes, you may do this, as long as no re-heating of the refrigerated portions will be required before serving them. Others say you should only add the supplements directly to one or two daily feedings immediately before you serve each one of them.

If you've already added certain supplements to the remaining servings for the day, it may not hurt to refrigerate them, but re-heating those previously refrigerated portions could definitely destroy the nutritional value of anything you've already added. And since some supplements specifically state on the bottle that they shouldn't be refrigerated ("store only in a cool dry place" or "do not refrigerate"), this advice would probably apply, whether the supplements were kept in the bottle or mixed in with the food.

If you're preparing a large batch of food to last for several days, and some of it will be frozen, then it's probably wisest to add supplements to the defrosted portions just before serving them.

If you can't add supplements to the total day's amount of food, should you put all of them into the first serving of the day?

It may be better not to try adding the entire day's supply of all vitamins, minerals and nutritional supplements to only a single serving. If your pet doesn't eat the entire serving and you have to throw some of it out, she won't have received all of the nutrients from the supplements that were mixed in with that meal. And it may be even better to divide the nutritional supplements for the day and mix half of that amount in with each of the two daily feedings so that your pet is more likely to absorb all of the nutrients at each meal. However, if you know your pet will always eat the whole bowl of food at one time, it's ok to go ahead and add all of the supplements at once.

Feeding nutritional supplements and oils

If any of the nutritional supplements you want your pet to take come in either capsule or tablet form, there's an easy way to assure that your pet gets the full dose. Simply wrap the capsule or tablet in a small amount of moist food and feed it by hand as if it's a special treat. This works for the majority of pets and may be better than using cheese or peanut butter for pets with certain types of health challenges.

When you're giving things like vitamin E oil, flaxseed oil, or supplements in powdered form, instead of mixing them in with the total amount of food for that meal, try mixing them into a smaller portion of the food which you serve first to be certain that all of it is consumed. Even these items can be put into empty gelatin capsules, wrapped with a little moist food and served as a special treat if necessary.

Recipe Suggestions

Arthritis diet for dogs

This diet is also recommended for loss of energy and weight management.

Ingredients:

1 cup brown rice
1 cup barley
1 cup carrots
1 cup spinach
½ cup lentils
½ cup celery
¼ cup parsley
1 cup lamb or beef heart
1 garlic clove
4 to 8 cups filtered or distilled water

Directions:

Combine all ingredients in a large pot. Bring to a boil, then simmer for 1¼ hours. Keep pot covered. Stir every 15 minutes. Add water if needed. Feed this diet for one month or until you see significant improvement.

Arthritis diet for cats

Ingredients:

1 cup protein (raw ground beef or chicken, or lightly cooked liver - all organic)
½ cup grated vegetables (raw is best)
½ cup complex carbohydrates (cooked millet, quinoa, buckwheat, barley or brown rice)

Directions:

Combine raw protein, raw veggies and cooked grain.
Add a multi vitamin/mineral supplement, *plus:*

- Vitamin C - 250 mg
- Vitamin E - 100 IU
- Vitamin A - 5,000 IU (from fish liver oil)

Once a week add Vitamin D - 400 IU
This diet may be fed on a continual basis.

Diabetic diet for dogs

Ingredients:

½ cup raw ground chuck or organic chicken
½ cup raw liver
½ cup cooked brown rice, oatmeal, or millet; or ½ cup raw oat bran soaked in water for at least 48 hours
¼ cup finely grated raw zucchini or carrot
¼ teaspoon grated garlic
Vegetable broth, kombu broth or parsley tea to moisten

Directions:

Cook the grain and lightly heat the broth or tea. Then combine all of the ingredients in a food processor and blend.
When the mixture is cool, add the following, gently mixing them in by hand:
Vitamin/mineral supplement
1 teaspoon chopped alfalfa sprouts
1 drop stevia extract or 1 teaspoon stevia tea.
Divide recipe into five separate feedings per day.

Diabetic diet for cats

Ingredients:

1 large raw egg (organic if possible)
½ cup creamed cottage cheese
½ cup cooked brown rice or other grain
1 tablespoon grated or chopped vegetables
1 teaspoon chopped alfalfa sprouts
Vegetable broth, parsley tea, or dill seed tea to moisten
1/16 teaspoon of potassium chloride (salt substitute)
1 drop stevia extract, or 1 teaspoon stevia tea
Multi-vitamin/mineral supplement
250 units of vitamin C

Directions:

Cook the grain and lightly heat the vegetable broth, parsley tea, or dill seed tea. Combine the first five ingredients in a blender or food processor. Add the broth or tea to the blended ingredients. Allow mixture to cool a little bit. Then add the last four ingredients and mix by hand. Feed three to five small meals a day.

Once a day add:

- 100 units vitamin E

Once a week add:

- 10,000 units vitamin A
- 400 units vitamin D by puncturing the capsules and adding the contents to the food

Pancreatitis diet for dogs

Ingredients:

3 cups chicken broth (homemade if possible)

¼ cup tomato juice (organic if possible, and _not_ V8 which is too high in sodium)

2 cups cooked grain (brown rice, quinoa, or barley)

1 cup raw peas

2 organic eggs (separate the whites and the yolks)

1½ cups organic raw liver cut in pieces

½ cup raw carrot or zucchini finely grated in a food processor

1 tablespoon bone meal

Vitamin C (amount depends on animal's weight)

Directions:

Combine broth, tomato juice, cooked grain, peas, and egg *whites* in a pan. Simmer for 3 minutes. Turn off heat and add raw liver pieces. Cover and let cool. Add raw grated vegetables, raw egg *yolks* and bone meal. Blend everything in a food processor. Add divided doses of Vitamin C and any other nutritional supplements before serving. Serve four times a day.

Pancreatitis diet for cats

This diet is high in B vitamins, anti-stress vitamins, protein and calcium. It's low in fat and easily digested.

Ingredients:

3 cups home made chicken broth simmered with ¼ cup tomato juice (no added salt)

2 cups cooked grain of your choice

1 cup raw peas

2 organic eggs (separate the whites and yolks)

1½ cups organic raw liver cut in pieces

½ cup finely grated raw carrot or zucchini
1 tablespoon bone meal or calcium gluconate

Directions:

Combine broth, cooked grain, raw peas and egg *whites* in a pan. Simmer for 3 minutes. Turn off heat and add organic raw liver pieces. Cover and let cool. Add raw egg *yolks*, raw vegetables, and bone meal. Blend in a blender or food processor. Store measured half-cup portions in freezer. Thaw as needed. Add any other nutritional supplements before serving. Serve ½ cup size servings 4 times a day.

Renal (kidney) diet for dogs

These are low-protein, low-phosphorus, high-potassium, normal sodium diets suitable for a medium size dog of about 20 pounds.

Recipe #1- Egg and Potato Diet

Ingredients:

1 large egg, cooked
3 cups potatoes, skin left on, sliced and boiled (sweet potato can be substituted here)
1 tablespoon chicken broth with fat
500-600 milligrams of calcium (buy tablets if necessary and crush them)
Multi-vitamin tablet

Directions:

Combine cooked egg, boiled potatoes and broth. Add calcium and multi-vitamin before serving.

Recipe #2 - Chicken and Potato Diet

Ingredients:

¼ cup cooked chicken (white breast meat is best)
3 cups potatoes, skin left on, sliced and boiled (sweet potato can be substituted here)
2 tablespoons chicken broth with fat
500-600 milligrams of calcium
Multi-vitamin tablet

Directions:

Combine cooked chicken, boiled potatoes and chicken broth. Add calcium and multi-vitamin before serving.

Recipe #3 - Beef and Potato Diet

Ingredients:

2 ounces ground beef (organic if fed raw; otherwise store bought and cooked)
3 cups potatoes, skin left on, sliced and boiled (sweet potato can be substituted here)
2 tablespoons of chicken broth with fat
500-600 milligrams of calcium
Multiple vitamin tablet

Directions:

Combine the beef, boiled potatoes and chicken broth. Add calcium and multi-vitamin before serving.

Recipe #4 - Egg and Tapioca Diet

Ingredients:

3 hard boiled eggs
2 cups tapioca cooked
1 tablespoon chicken broth with fat
500-600 milligrams of calcium
Multiple vitamin tablet

Directions:

Combine hard boiled eggs, cooked tapioca and chicken broth. Add calcium and multi-vitamin before serving.

You may use the following substitutions in the Egg and Tapioca Diet:

- Beef instead of hard boiled eggs - use 4 ounces cooked lean ground beef
- Chicken instead of hard boiled eggs - use ½ cup cooked chicken breast
- Egg Whites Only - prepare 3 hard boiled eggs but use only the whites

Recipe # 5 - Eggs and Rice Diet

Ingredients:

1 large hard boiled egg
2 cups of cooked brown rice
1 tablespoon of chicken broth with fat

500-600 milligrams of calcium
Multi-vitamin tablet

Directions:

Combine hard boiled eggs, cooked brown rice and chicken broth. Add calcium and multi-vitamin before serving. (*Note*: You may use either 1 whole egg, or the whites of 3 hard boiled eggs, in the Egg and Rice Diet.)

Renal (kidney) diet for cats

A diet for cats with kidney disease needs to be high in complex carbohydrates with proteins that are carefully balanced. It should also include a couple of drops of golden seal elixir (not tincture) a day and plenty of distilled water.

Ingredients:

1 cup cooked pureed barley flakes and/or baby food creamed corn
½ cup lightly boiled or broiled chicken or beef, or 1 raw organic egg yolk, or cooked egg white.
¼ cup chopped or finely grated raw vegetables or vegetable juice (include carrots, zucchini, and alfalfa sprouts)
2 teaspoons of soft butter
Vitamin/Mineral Supplement

Directions:

Blend all ingredients and store in refrigerator until ready to serve. Bring to room temperature and add vitamin/mineral supplement before serving. Because nutrients tend to be eliminated quickly in the urine, feed patients with kidney disease four or more times a day.

Urinary tract and bladder conditions—diet for dogs and cats

Ingredients:

3 cups filtered or distilled water
1 cup brown rice or millet (not the instant variety)
½ cup boneless, skinless chicken, cubed (organic)
2 raw egg yolks (use organic eggs, if possible)
2 tablespoons minced parsley
2 tablespoons grated asparagus
1 tablespoon sesame oil (unrefined)
Multi-vitamin/mineral supplement

Directions:

Cook brown rice or millet well with 2½ cups of water for about 45 minutes. With remaining water, cook chicken slightly for 5 minutes. Add raw egg yolks, finely chopped raw vegetables, and the oil to the cooked brown rice or millet. Add slightly cooked chicken to this mixture. Add supplements to cooled mixture.

The parsley and asparagus act as gentle diuretics, helping flush impurities out of the system. You can also use nettles and dandelion leaves. Since nutrients are washed out quickly in the urine, it's a good idea to feed three or four times a day.

Chapter 9

Healthy Recipes For Pets With Other Special Needs

The recipes in this chapter are also designed for small breed dogs weighing up to about 20 pounds. Consequently, the quantities in each recipe will need to be significantly increased for larger dogs, or the serving sizes will need to be decreased for very small dogs.

The total number of meals you'll be able to serve from a single recipe will depend on how much food your pet needs to eat in a day. This usually depends on an individual pet's weight and appetite. As a rule of thumb, feed two servings each day unless otherwise indicated in the recipe.

If you're adding vitamins, minerals or other nutritional supplements to any of these recipes, you'll find detailed information about how to do this wisely in the introduction to the previous chapter, "**Recipes Designed for Pets with Major Health Challenges**."

Recipe suggestions

Anti-tapeworm diet for dogs

Ingredients:

2 cups canned pumpkin
½ cup wheat germ
¼ cup blackstrap molasses

Directions:

Mix ingredients together and then mix them in with the pet's regular food. For small dogs, use 1 to 2 tablespoons per meal; for large dogs, use ¼ cup. Give once a day for two days. After a couple of days, the dogs should pass the tapeworms.

Anti-tapeworm diet for cats:

Ingredients:

½ cup soaked oats (rolled oats soaked in water for 24 hours)
2 tablespoons cod, haddock, or halibut simmered one minute in a small amount of water
Garlic, raw, crushed (the size of a pea)
Vitamin/Mineral Supplement

Directions:

Mix ingredients together and feed twice a day, while at the same time treating with medicine to kill the worms.

Healthy skin - diet for dogs

Ingredients:

1½ cups brown rice
1 cup barley
1 cup carrots
1 cup beets
½ cup beet tops
½ cup spinach
1 cup chicken livers or giblets
1 garlic clove
¼ teaspoon sage
4 to 6 cups water

Directions:

Combine ingredients in a large pot. Bring to a boil. Simmer for 1¼ hours. Keep pot covered; stir every 15 minutes; add water if needed.

Healthy skin - diet recommendations for cats

Allergies and toxins show up in a cat's skin as bald patches, scabs, inflammation, oiliness, bad odor or dandruff. This may happen for a variety of reasons. The diet should immediately be changed to a raw food diet without any artificial chemicals or additives.
Follow these simple directions:

1. Fast on chicken broth and/or teas for 1-3 days.
2. Feed a raw food diet using raw meats, raw vegetables, and soaked oats. Use alkalizing vegetables such as garlic, kelp, kombu, seaweed, carrots, celery, zucchini and string beans. (See

Chapter 2, **"Some Wholesome Alternatives,"** for detailed instructions.)

3. Remove all food in between meals. No crunchies and no treats either.

4. Add vitamins, minerals and other nutritional supplements to food.

5. Add ¼ teaspoon skin and coat oil supplement for cats from health food store.

6. Give 5 mg zinc once a day for two weeks; then decrease to 2 mg a day. This strengthens the skin and helps the body process out toxins.

7. Because it's possible that skin problems may result from being depressed or bored, add three drops of Bach Flower Rescue Remedy to the cat's food or water.

8. Bathe every one to four weeks using natural preparations for the skin.

9. Stimulate the flow of blood in the small capillaries by grooming or massaging vigorously once a day.

Low calorie diet for dogs and cats

Ingredients:

3 cups water

½ cup rice or 1 cup rolled oats, barley or cornmeal (if your pet isn't allergic to corn)

3 tablespoons soy flour (or substitute 1 raw egg for the soy flour, but add the egg only after the cereal mixture has cooled to room temperature)

½ cup bran

½ cup powdered wheat germ

¼ cup powdered skim milk

¼ lb raw lean ground beef or fish

1 or 2 oz raw beef liver

2 tablespoons of vegetables

1 teaspoon kelp

1 tablespoon brewers yeast

1 teaspoon bone meal

½ teaspoon cod liver oil and ½ teaspoon wheat germ oil mixed together (or 1 teaspoon of either oil used alone)

Directions:

Boil 3 cups of water, add cereal grains and soy flour and simmer covered. When almost done, add bran, powdered skim milk, and powdered wheat germ. Stir, add a little more water if necessary, and finish cooking. Uncover and let mixture cool.

Add meat, liver, vegetables, kelp and brewers yeast to cooled cereal/soy flour mixture, then blend all of these ingredients in a food processor.

Mix bone meal in with the cod liver oil and wheat germ oil to dissolve it well. Add this mixture, plus a multi-vitamin/mineral supplement, and any additional nutritional supplements to the food mixture just before serving. Serve four times a day.

If a pet's coat begins to look a little dull, add a teaspoon or two of olive oil or flaxseed oil.

Low-fat, high-fiber diet for dogs and cats

Ingredients:

4 ounces lean ground beef
2 cups cooked carrots
½ cup dry cottage cheese
2 cups green beans
1 teaspoon bone meal
½ teaspoon garlic powder

Directions:

Cook beef and drain off any fat. Cook carrots. Mix all ingredients together. Feed two servings each day.

Satin balls

This is a recipe to fatten up your dog, get momma dogs to eat and produce milk, or put a "glow" on show dogs. Satin Balls are a high carbohydrate, high fat snack. For this reason, they're definitely *not* recommended for overweight dogs or those suffering from yeast infections. Both of the Satin Ball recipes below may also be used for cats.

Ingredients:

1 lb raw ground beef (high % fat)
1 cup Total cereal (in the blue box as of this writing)
1 cup uncooked old fashioned oatmeal
1 raw egg

3 tablespoons wheat germ
1 package Knox unflavored gelatin
2 tablespoons vegetable oil
2 tablespoons unsulfured molasses
Pinch of salt

Directions:

Mix all ingredients thoroughly and shape into serving-size meatballs or patties.

It's better to feed raw, but if you like, you can cook the meat briefly in a pan.

Freeze the Satin Balls in individual serving sizes. Thaw for a couple of hours before serving, or submerge bag in hot water for a few moments to defrost, then serve.

Alternate recipe for satin balls

Ingredients:

2 lbs raw ground beef
½ pint whipping cream
½ box old fashioned oatmeal
½ of a large jar of *natural* peanut butter
12 egg yolks
1 pint cottage cheese (use the 4%, not the low fat!)
¼ cup molasses

Directions:

Mix all ingredients together & shape into small balls.

Milk replacement for newborn puppies and kittens

Ingredients:

2 cups whole milk, or 1 cup evaporated milk and 1 cup water
1 raw egg yolk
¼ cup brewer's yeast
2 tablespoons cream, or 1 tablespoon unsaturated oil
½ teaspoon bone meal

Directions:

Mix ingredients together well. For puppies, add a crushed vitamin formulated especially for them. For kittens, add crushed vitamins formulated for them. Also for kittens, if the supplement does not contain Taurine, add 100 mg of Taurine as well.

Warm the mixture just to the animal's body temperature and feed by bottle. (Remember that an animal's body temperature is normally around 101-102 degrees Fahrenheit.) Feed puppies or kittens only enough at each feeding to enlarge the abdomen slightly, but not distend it.

After each feeding, gently massage the belly, and swab the genital and anal area with a warm moistened hand towel. This will stimulate proper urination and defecation.

You can introduce solids at about 4 weeks of age by using less liquid and preparing this same formula as a thin paste instead of as a liquid.

Feeding schedule for puppies and kittens

Age	Weight	Frequency
0-2 weeks	4-8 oz.	Every 2 hours
3 weeks	8-10 oz.	Every 3 hours
4-5 weeks	10-24 oz.	Every 4 hours
6 weeks	2 lbs. or more	3 times a day

Weaning from bottle to soft food for puppies and kittens

Sometimes we find ourselves with very young animals who have been taken away from their mothers too soon for a variety of reasons. Since mom isn't around, it's up to us to help them learn to transition from formula to solid food. Here's some help.

Ingredients:

1 jar lamb, beef or chicken baby food (*no* onion, onion powder, onion salt or added salt)
3 teaspoons vegetable baby food - carrot, squash or pumpkin

2 teaspoons uncooked baby food cereal flakes - creamed barley
1 organic raw egg yolk or ½ teaspoon butter
½ teaspoon brewer's yeast
Liquid vitamins and calcium based on pet's weight
Distilled water sufficient to mix

Directions:

Mix all ingredients to a soft consistency and feed every four hours, or four to five times a day for the first week. Then, depending on how old the animal is, and how well it's eating, you can decrease the frequency. This is good for both dogs and cats. Puppies and kittens need to be fed three times a day from six weeks of age until they're six months old, and then twice a day until they're eight months old. After that once or twice a day is fine.

The above formula might also be good to feed to a very old cat if you use a much larger quantity of vitamins and minerals. Remember, as animals age, they need less protein because they're less active.

Diet for older dogs and cats

Older animals may need less protein, but it needs to be a high quality protein. Many conditions associated with old age, such as arthritis, heart problems, coughs, kidney failure, bad teeth and even some tumors, could be prevented if only pets were fed a highly nutritious diet throughout their lives. Some conditions can be improved by switching to a higher quality diet even when a pet is older.

Ingredients

½ cup of brown rice
1 egg
½ lb lean raw meat or fish
1 oz raw liver
2 tablespoons chopped vegetables
1 tablespoon diced parsley or a combination of fresh herbs
1 teaspoon of crushed garlic
1 tablespoon olive oil or flaxseed oil

Directions:

Cook rice over low heat as directed. Once cooked, add the egg to the hot rice until egg has cooked. Once cooled, mix the raw meats, vegetables, parsley, garlic and oil into the mixture.

Add all of the following supplements before feeding:

- 1 tablespoon bran
- 1 tablespoon wheat germ
- 1 tablespoon brewers yeast
- ½ tablespoon lecithin
- 1 teaspoon bone meal
- 1 teaspoon kelp
- 1 teaspoon alfalfa powder
- 1 teaspoon cod liver oil and wheat germ oil mixed
- 1/8 teaspoon chelated magnesium or Epsom salt

Food allergy diet

Ingredients:

½ cup brown rice
1½ cups water
¼ lb raw chicken, turkey or lamb (only one of them) for dogs; ½ lb for cats
¼ cup grated carrots
1 teaspoon kelp or trace mineral supplement
½ teaspoon bonemeal

Directions:

Cook rice in 1½ cups of boiling water. Mix all ingredients together. Feed for two weeks.

Some of the allergy problems may seem to get worse for awhile, but don't despair, the diet is working. After allergy symptoms stop, you can experiment with different meats and add other ingredients to the recipe, but be sure to change or add only one new item at a time. If the allergy symptoms flare up again, you'll know which food is the cause and needs to be avoided.

A word about reactions to foods

Reactions to foods may be classified as a sensitivity, an intolerance or an actual allergy.

Food *sensitivities* usually occur when there are hormonal imbalances.

Food *intolerance* may involve one or more ingredients, or a combination of one or more ingredients. The offending substances may include wheat or rice, poor sources of protein, or additives used in commercial pet foods.

Food *allergies* often translate into skin disorders, intestinal upset, vomiting and diarrhea. In some instances, they may be related to endocrine-immune imbalances. Although it's not very common, food *allergies* can even account for catastrophic episodes where pets may die.

In some animals, a small amount of the offending food can trigger a bad reaction, even if the food is organically grown.

When a diet is made up of inferior ingredients, which are sometimes used in cheaper commercial pet foods, food sensitivities, intolerances or allergies may become more pronounced. Other signs of reactions to foods may include wanting to eat almost non-stop and excessive defecation.

The most common foods that may cause reactions in pets are listed below:

Foods that may cause reactions

Dogs:	Cats:
Wheat	Wheat
Milk	Milk and Dairy Products
Eggs	Eggs
Brewer's Yeast	Brewer's Yeast
Corn and Corn Oil	Corn and Corn Oil
Pork	Pork
Lamb	Fish
Chicken	Chicken
Turkey	Turkey
Beef and Beef By-Products	Beef
Soybeans	
Rice	

Some alternatives to use in place of foods on the above lists, especially for dogs, are: duck and potatoes, venison and potatoes, or rabbit and potatoes. Cats would require higher levels of duck, venison or rabbit, but only minimal amounts of potatoes.

Most animals are not sensitive to potatoes, but if they are, then any other complex carbohydrate could be used instead. This would include brown rice, millet, barley, quinoa, etc.

To prevent an animal from acquiring an intolerance to a particular food, gradually rotate the meats and grains every four to six months.

Once a pet develops a sensitivity to one or more foods or additives, his or her immune cells retain the memory of that particular offender, so it's unreasonable to think we can wean a pet off those foods or additives for awhile, and then re-introduce them at a later date.

For those of you who need to do further research on allergies and how endocrine-immune imbalances may be a major cause of multiple chronic illnesses in pets, look for the book *Pets At Risk*, co-authored by Alfred J. Plechner, DVM, and Martin Zucker.

Chapter 10

The Art of Using Herbs as Medicine

Herbs are not only beneficial for treating physical problems, but they're also very effective for treating a pet's emotional and behavioral problems.

My work with animals has shown me over and over again that they experience complex mental and emotional activity, and that they, too, feel many of the same stresses and anxieties people go through. When this happens, the effects of those feelings will eventually show up in their bodies or in their behavior.

But many animals will respond very well to herbs, *if you are consistent about using them,* and *if you will give them sufficient time to work.* Herbs are a form of food, so they don't work as quickly as most medications do. Unlike many drugs, however, herbs are relatively safe to take. But the key to using them is consistency.

Herbal healing, or the art of using plants as medicine, is one of the oldest healing traditions. The medicinal use of plants goes back for generations and only began to be replaced after pharmaceutical companies became prevalent. Yet, there's a definite place for both herbal preparations *and* pharmaceutical medications.

Your pet may require a specific pharmaceutical medication in an emergency, or when an illness is so far advanced that it requires strong doses of medicine to control the disease or condition. However, in most other cases, you may find that the natural healing benefits of certain herbs and plants are very beneficial for your pets, and, when used correctly, they don't have the side effects that many medications do.

Animals need greens for nutrition and proper digestion. Often, they even know intuitively which plants will help them medicinally when they aren't feeling well. If a particular plant grows in the area, they'll intentionally seek it out all by themselves.

For most of our pets, however, grass is about the only green substance they have access to. Everyone has seen pets eat grass on occasion and seem to feel better afterwards, once the grass has caused them to empty their stomachs of whatever was bothering them.

But what are some other herbs and plants you might find useful for your pet?

I'm not an expert, and I can't explain the use of each and every one of them, but I have compiled a reference list to help guide you in the right direction. You should do your own in-depth research before starting to use herbs for your pets.

It's important to be aware that cats may respond differently to some herbs than dogs will. For that reason, it's wise to check with a professional herbalist, or with someone who knows the benefits, characteristics and interactions of herbs before you implement treatments on your own.

The same caution holds true when you want to use several different herbs at the same time. While it's sometimes beneficial to use multiple herbs together, if they have similar properties or actions, herbs used in combination may produce effects which are much stronger than the effects of the same herbs used individually.

Please remember that the information I'm providing in these five chapters about herbs for healing purposes is only an overview, and should be regarded only as a *general* guideline. You should consult with a holistic veterinarian or knowledgeable herbalist to determine what will be the best and safest way to treat your pet.

Before we look at a list of herbs and their potential uses, let's become acquainted with (1) those herbs that should be used only with the appropriate cautions, and (2) those herbs which should *not* be used at all.

Herbs to be used with caution

The following herbs should be used with great caution for any animal, or used only under the guidance of a trained herbologist:

- **Juniper Berries** should not be used long-term because they irritate the kidneys and urinary tract;
- **Uva Ursi** has a strong astringent action and should not be used long-term because it also irritates the kidneys and urinary tract;
- **Horsetail** used long-term can elevate blood pressure;

- **Licorice** can lead to water retention and raise blood pressure – best not to use on a long-term basis;
- **Ginkgo** should not be used with veterinarian-prescribed heart medications or blood thinners;
- **Hawthorne Berry** is not for use with veterinarian-prescribed heart medications or blood thinners; however both Hawthorne Berry and Ginkgo, if used correctly, can help reduce the need for some medications;
- **Goldenseal, Barberry, and Oregon Grape Root** have strong astringent action – best for short-term use only because they can reduce the amount of beneficial bacteria if used for too long a time.

The following herbs should *never* be given to cats internally:

- **White Willow Bark**
- **Meadowsweet**
- **Mistletoe**
- **Pennyroyal** (check for this herb as a flea collar ingredient)
- **Rue**
- **Wormwood**

Herbs and their possible uses

ALFALFA

Stimulates digestion and appetite; helps with urinary problems; good source of vitamin K.

ALOE VERA

This gel has been used for centuries to stimulate healing for burns, sunburns, and wounds. It also relieves skin ulcers and inflammation. As a drying agent, it's useful for healing ulcerous sores. Use it externally by applying pure fresh gel from the plant to the wound, sore, or hot spot, or use a high quality aloe vera gel obtained from a health food store.

Internally, aloe vera is often used as an herb for problems like constipation, appendicitis, colitis, abdominal pain, to facilitate digestion, aid in blood and lymphatic circulation, and to improve liver, kidney and gall bladder functions.

Aloe vera can also be used internally to help detoxify a pet. This may be beneficial for a pet who's suffering from skin problems, or needs to be cleansed after using chemically based drugs.

ARNICA

Has anti-inflammatory properties; relieves the pain of bruises, hyperextensions, sprains, arthritis, bursitis, rheumatism and inflammation; can be made into a tea or tincture and applied as a compress, or added to a massage oil; should not be applied to an open wound; not for internal use.

ASTRAGALUS

Used to treat anxiety and fatigue; heals, repairs, and supports the entire body by increasing stamina and building resistance to disease and infection; its diuretic properties help the kidneys and urinary tract; also helpful for conditions relating to spleen, lungs and blood.

BLACK WALNUT EXTRACT

Kills and expels worms and helps with fungal infections; an effective treatment for diarrhea; helps to repel mosquitoes from animals when they take it internally.

BOSWELLIA

Has been shown to have anti-inflammatory effects so it's often used for conditions in which inflammation plays a part like arthritis, inflammatory bowel disease, Crohn's disease, and asthma. It may also help the liver and relieve brain inflammation.

BURDOCK

Cleanses the blood and helps to detoxify the body; is useful for skin disorders; lowers blood sugar levels; can also be used as a kidney tonic and to increase immunity. Burdock is an ingredient in Essiac tea which is often recommended for animals with cancer and other serious illnesses.

CALENDULA

Can be used externally to disinfect wounds, help heal the skin, and treat sores, burns and fungal infections; can be used internally for gastrointestinal disorders, stomach cramps, ulcers, inflammation of the large intestine, blood or bacteria in the urine, fluid retention, viral infections, liver disorders, and worms.

CARAWAY

Helps to stimulate the appetite and ease occasional bouts of diarrhea and upset stomach.

CASCARA SAGRADA

Acts as a laxative to help with constipation; helps improve digestion.

CATNIP

Helps relieve muscle spasms, colds, fevers, diarrhea, and gas in cats. In general cats love to smell it, eat it and roll around in fresh or dried catnip. They may purr, meow, roll over and leap, much the way they do when they're in heat. Catnip has an interesting dual action. It may act as a stimulant in cats when it's sniffed, but it will also act as a sedative if swallowed.

CHAMOMILE

Used as a calming agent, antispasmodic, aromatic and stimulant. It soothes both mind and body, helps prevent infection, heals wounds, relieves indigestion and ulcers, relaxes the nerves, alleviates inflammation and skin irritations, prevents insomnia and relieves both headaches and muscle cramps. Taken internally as a tea, it can help calm anxious, clingy pets, and also relieve nausea, indigestion and insomnia. Externally as a tea, it can be useful for treating conjunctivitis and skin problems.

COMFREY

Used externally, comfrey speeds the healing of wounds and even broken bones. It's also useful for digestive disorders, urinary tract infections, diarrhea, hernias, hemorrhoids and ulcers.

CORNSILK

Soothes kidney and bladder inflammation and incontinence.

DANDELION

Acts as a tonic for the digestive tract and as a blood cleanser and diuretic. Add fresh leaves to food for improved liver function. Also effective in the treatment of arthritis.

DEVIL'S CLAW ROOT

Helpful for the treatment of arthritis, rheumatism, and lower back pain; effective in reducing inflammation and improving range of motion; a good stimulant for the lymph system; can be used as a detoxifying herb for the whole body.

DILL

Used as a stomach-soothing agent for cats; can help relieve nausea and flatulence, especially when triggered by a sudden change in diet.

ECHINACEA

Fights bacterial and viral infections; has been described as a "super herb" because of its ability to help the body fight infections by supporting the immune system. Interestingly, dogs with allergies have sometimes benefited from this herb.

EYEBRIGHT

Can be used internally as a tea, or externally as an eye wash; useful for cats who have an eye that is weepy, red and irritated; may help clear up this type of eye problem.

FENUGREEK

Often used as an appetizer; can be used to help gain weight and condition the body.

FEVERFEW

Helps prevent migraine headaches and, when added to horse and dog meals, often relieves arthritis pain and increases mobility; used also for psoriasis and stress.

FLAXSEED OIL

An excellent source of omega-3 fatty acids (the good fats which help reduce the primary artery blockers - cholesterol and triglycerides); helpful for preventing blood clots.

GARLIC

Regarded as another "wonder herb" for all of its various benefits for both humans and animals. Many of these benefits are already well known. For pets, garlic can help support the digestive system, and can also act as a natural flea repellent. Garlic changes the "flavor" of your pet's blood, and although animals love the pungent taste of garlic, fleas don't! Please be careful, though. Small amounts of garlic are always beneficial, but it should never be used in large amounts, even for healthy pets. Some pets may be allergic to it, and if a dog or cat has been diagnosed with anemia, they should not be eating garlic at all. (See Chapter 6, **"Foods All Pets Should Avoid,"** for more information.)

GINKGO

Ginkgo is an anti-aging herb which acts on two major systems of the body: the nervous system and the cardiovascular system. In animals, senile dementia associated with Alzheimer's-like symptoms is referred to as cognitive dysfunction or dimming mind syndrome. Ginkgo enhances both long-term and short-term memory in puppies and older animals alike. This popular herb improves circulation and has beneficial antioxidant activity. Studies also indicate that ginkgo is often effective as a treatment for dizziness and vertigo, as well as age-related hearing and vision loss.

GINGER

Prescribed in China for colds, flu, coughs, respiratory problems and kidney disease, ginger was also discovered to successfully relieve nausea. It improves circulation and digestion. To help pets who suffer from motion sickness, give 1 capsule per 25 pounds of body weight half an hour before leaving home. As an alternative, you can use a few drops of ginger root extract. If this isn't effective, the dose may need to be increased. Fresh ginger can also be added to pet food in small amounts as a digestive tonic and to prevent flatulence.

GINSENG

Boosts the immune system, improves stamina and endurance, reduces stress, and can help improve performance; trainers may use this herb to help animals train and compete.

GOLDENSEAL

A beneficial herb for both internal and external use. Internally, it has strong anti-bacterial properties which have been shown to kill a variety of germs, such as those that cause yeast infections, as well as various parasites like tapeworms and giardia. It may also be capable of activating white blood cells, making the body more capable of fighting infection. Its ability to counteract microbes makes it useful in conditions like urinary tract infections and infectious diarrhea. Externally it can be used as an anti-inflammatory and antiseptic to clean wounds, alleviate skin infections and treat conjunctivitis.

GRAPEFRUIT SEED EXTRACT/CITRUS SEED EXTRACT

Slows cancer cell growth and is a very powerful antioxidant; effective in treating parasites, viruses, ear infections, gum disease, fungal infections, diarrhea and drug-resistant bacteria. Cats, however, may not respond favorably to citrus products.

GREEN TEA

The green variety of tea contains flavonoids and polyphenols, which are a type of flavonoid that may be a more powerful antioxidant than vitamins C and E. Green tea is oxidized for a shorter period of time than black tea. Many practitioners don't think the black variety has the same health benefits as those found in green tea.

HAWTHORN

Used mainly as a cardiac tonic to treat organic and functional heart troubles. Also useful as a diuretic, astringent, and tonic. Both the flowers and berries have astringent properties. It's useful as a diuretic, for cases of dropsy, and for kidney trouble.

HOPS

A diuretic, stimulant, alterative (something that brings about gradual beneficial changes), and astringent herb that promotes digestion by increasing the flow of bile; also effective for treating parasitic worms; in tincture form, it helps lower blood sugar and has an anti-diabetic effect.

HORSETAIL

Stimulates the metabolic processes that repair bones and connective tissue.

KELP AND OTHER SEAWEEDS

In addition to correcting mineral deficiencies, kelp and other seaweeds contain alginates that soothe and cleanse the digestive tract while preventing the absorption of toxic metals. Seaweeds also protect against heart and kidney disease and improve glandular function. They can promote rapid hair growth and correct pigmentation, making black fur and noses blacker.

LICORICE

Beneficial for respiratory system, digestion and adrenal glands; used for cough, bronchial congestion, asthma, and acute gastritis; also useful for stress and exhaustion.

MARSHMALLOW

Useful in treating gastrointestinal problems, particularly inflammatory and ulcerative conditions, spasms, colitis, diarrhea and constipation. It also has expectorant properties, which make it ideal for treating dry coughs, congestion, and respiratory disorders. Caution: Marshmallow has the potential to exacerbate hypoglycemia, so check with your veterinarian before giving marshmallow to an animal with low blood sugar.

MICROALGAE (Chlorella, Spirulina, Blue-Green Algae)

These are among the world's most widespread and popular herbs, but not every strain of algae is edible. The ones used in food supplements must be non-toxic and rich in chlorophyll, amino acids, vitamins, minerals and protein. You can find these in almost every quality pet supplement.

MILK THISTLE

An amazing herb for both humans and dogs! Milk Thistle has been used to support and maintain liver function. The liver is a food processor, a storehouse for nutrients, and a factory that makes hormones and other substances. It's also a filter that removes toxins from the blood. Feed milk thistle to any pet who has been fed a commercial diet, been exposed to chemical pesticides like garden sprays or flea and tick repellents, or who has elevated liver enzymes, or can benefit from regular liver support.

MULLEIN

Beneficial for respiratory system problems; acts as an anti-inflammatory, antispasmodic, expectorant, astringent, and as a soothing nerve tonic (sometimes called a soothing nervine); alleviates congestion, is a great painkiller and soporific (sleeping aid); also soothes and strengthens the intestines and kidneys; can be added to any pet food, fresh or dried.

NETTLE

Can help to stimulate a dog's appetite by acting like a tonic; is also an expectorant, antispasmodic, and alterative (something that brings about gradual beneficial changes); used in animals with respiratory problems, allergies, asthma, arthritis, skin and coat disorders, and conditions involving the kidneys or urinary tract; the powdered form of the common stinging nettle is often used in cases of flaky or scaly skin conditions and for hair loss where bald patches appear; can also help hair to grow back.

OATS

Helps with nervous system, as in epilepsy, tremors, twitching and paralysis.

PARSLEY

The root can be used as a diuretic, laxative, and eyewash. Eaten raw or taken as a tea, the leaves can help alleviate bladder problems and freshen breath. Parsley has a high vitamin content including vitamins A, B-Complex, and C, as well as iron, calcium and potassium.

PAU D'ARCO

Has powerful anti-fungal and immune building qualities; considered to be an analgesic, antioxidant, antiparasitic, antimicrobial, antifungal, antiviral, antibacterial, and anti-inflammatory; has anticancerous properties and can help stengthen a weakened immune system; useful for treating diabetes, allergies, liver disease and yeast infections; used for treating arthritis, tumors, polyps, warts, skin ulcerations, boils, dysentery, gastrointestinal problems, urinary tract infections, cancer and respiratory problems, fevers and infections; helps to alleviate pain; may help the body absorb nutrients as well as helping the body to eliminate wastes (laxative action).

PEPPERMINT

All members of the mint family are excellent for soothing digestive disturbances, including gas, indigestion, and colic. Also for other internal aches and pains. It's often given to pets orally as a tea or in tablet form. It can be inhaled by rubbing some peppermint tea on the chest area, or by using a drop of peppermint essential oil which has been *very well* diluted (80-90%) with some food grade or massage type mixing oil.

RED CLOVER BLOSSOM

Has sedative and antispasmodic properties; used as a blood-cleansing herb and a potent aid to detoxification.

ROSEMARY

This versatile antioxidant herb repels insects, relieves flatulence, and eases muscular and nerve pain. It helps ease the itch and dryness associated with eczema and soothes the soreness of arthritis.

SAGE

Has cleansing and astringent actions and antiseptic properties that are useful for healing infections.

SLIPPERY ELM

Soothes inflamed mucous membranes and is useful for treating diarrhea; also used internally for stomach ulcers, colitis, and coughs; can be used topically for wounds and abscesses.

ROSEHIPS

A great natural source of vitamin C that helps support a pet's immune system to fight off viral and bacterial infections.

ROSEMARY

An important antioxidant with bioactive ingredients which help prevent the breakdown of the chemical acetylcholine in the brain. A deficiency in acetylcholine is believed to be a contributing factor in senility in general and in Alzheimer's disease in particular.

TURMERIC

Turmeric is the yellow component of curry powder which stimulates the liver's bile production. This herb is a potent antioxidant. Turmeric is also heart healthy, acting as a blood thinner (which prevents clots) and it helps to prevent excess cholesterol accumulation.

VALERIAN ROOT

Calms and soothes the nerves, reducing tension and anxiety; best known as an aid to sleep; recommended for any pet suffering from stress, intestinal cramps, nervousness, restlessness, muscle spasm or bronchial spasms.

WORMWOOD

Gets rid of intestinal parasites; also has antiseptic, antispasmodic, and stimulant properties making it a tonic for the stomach and digestive tract; used as a tea or in capsule form.

YELLOW DOCK

Used extensively in the treatment of chronic skin complaints such as psoriasis; also a valuable remedy for constipation because it promotes the flow of bile and can act as a blood cleanser; useful for treating jaundice because it helps relieve congestion in the gall-bladder; can also be made into a tea and applied to cotton swabs to get rid of ear mites.

YUCCA

Reduces stress and swelling in the joints; a popular ingredient in arthritis blends for pets.

Ten favorite herbs for cats

Here's a list in alphabetical order of the top 10 favorite herbs for cats. Without a doubt, catnip rules as one of the most favored of the ten for felines because it adds zip and zest to their lives.

1.	**Burdock**	6.	**Echinacea**
2.	**Calendula**	7.	**Eyebright**
3.	**Caraway**	8.	**Parsley**
4.	**Catnip**	9.	**Rosemary**
5.	**Dill**	10.	**Valerian**

Ten favorite herbs for dogs

And here's a list in alphabetical order of the 10 favorite herbs for dogs:

1.	**Aloe vera**	7.	**Kelp**
2.	**Blackberry leaves** (applied for rashes or eczema)	8.	**Myrrh** (in combination with goldenseal can be given for colds and coughs)
3.	**Calendula**		
4.	**Chamomile**		
5.	**Echinacea**	9.	**Rosemary**
6.	**Goldenseal** (for skin diseases)	10.	**Witch hazel** (for bathing wounds)

* * *

As you can see, there are many herbal choices listed above for helping our pets, but there are still others with which you should also become familiar, so in the next chapter, we'll take a look at Ancient Indian (Ayurvedic) and Chinese Herbs.

Chapter 11

Ayurvedic and Chinese Herbs

While the herbs listed in the previous chapter are fairly well known in the Western world, many other healing herbs are also available to us, both for ourselves and for our pets. These herbs have successfully been used for centuries by the peoples of India and China.

A few of these herbal remedies have already come into common use, so you'll find them listed in both chapters.

Ayurvedic herbs

The Ayurvedic system of healing uses herbs for food and medicine to help restore balance in the body. This holistic healing system has been practiced in India for more than 5,000 years. The Sanskrit meaning of *ayu* is "life" and the meaning of *veda* is "knowing" or "science" so you might say that *Ayurveda* is "the science of life."

Ayurvedic treatments use a number of herbs which we consider to be traditional cooking spices, such as coriander, fennel, ginger, turmeric and black pepper. But there are also many other herbs used in Ayurveda which you might find useful. Following is a list of just a few of the many Ayurvedic herbs you may want to be aware of for your pets.

AMALAKI

Used to rebuild and maintain new tissues and increase red blood cell count; considered helpful for cleansing the mouth, strengthening the teeth, and nourishing the bones; a very high source of natural vitamin C; one of three herbs used in triphala, the primary Ayurvedic tonic for maintaining health.

ARJUNA

A well known cardiac tonic used in Ayurveda for a variety of heart conditions; used to lower blood pressure and heart rate; traditionally given to support circulation and oxygenation of all tissues; often combined with ashwagandha, brahmi and guggul in heart formulas.

ASHOKA

Believed to help maintain proper function of the female reproductive system; used in Ayurveda as a tonic for the uterus; may be particularly helpful for breeds, like bulldogs, who have a history of difficulty giving birth, or for animals who have suffered miscarriages.

ASHWAGANDHA

An Asian plant of the potato family, its roots have long been used to treat rheumatism, high blood pressure, immune dysfunction, and reduce inflammation. Ashwagandha has also traditionally been used for general debility and nerve exhaustion. It's said to regenerate the hormonal system, promote healing of tissues, and support sound sleep. It's also considered to be the primary adaptogenic Ayurvedic herb because it helps to build up the reserves necessary for handling stressful conditions. When used in combination with Boswellia, it's very beneficial for animals with arthritis. Ashwagandha is sometimes called the "Indian ginseng."

BACOPA

Assists in heightening mental acuity and supporting the body's ability to relax; used in formulas for mental exertion; animals with ADD or ADHD-like symptoms might benefit from taking this herb.

BHRINGARAJ

Considered helpful for loss of hair, loss of teeth, enlargement of the liver or spleen, chronic hepatitis, anemia and skin diseases; also available in oil form.

BHUMY AMALAKI

Provides very effective support for hepatitis C; is also used for numerous other conditions including blennorrhagia, colic, diabetes, dysentery, fever, tumors, jaundice, vaginitis and dyspepsia.

BIBITAKI

Used as a laxative to cleanse the bowels; one of three herbs used in triphala, the primary Ayurvedic tonic for maintaining health.

BITTER MELON

Has been shown to regulate the body's ability to process sugars; also see gymnema and chandraprabha for control of blood sugar levels.

BOSWELLIA

A potent anti-inflammatory shown to help relieve the stiffness and pain of arthritis. It supports healthy joints, shrinks inflamed tissues, and improves the blood supply to the affected area while repairing local blood vessels damaged by inflammation. Along with its cousin, guggul, Boswellia has many cholesterol and triglyceride lowering properties. Promising results were observed in patients with rheumatoid arthritis, chronic colitis, bronchial asthma and Crohn's disease. Usual dosage: for dogs up to 30 lbs, use 10 drops of liquid twice daily for each 10 pounds of body weight, or one 500 mg capsule or tablet twice daily; for dogs up to 60 lbs, use 500 mg three times daily; larger dogs may use 1,000 mg twice daily. This is one of the herbs that should definitely be given after feeding to prevent it from producing too much acidity in the stomach.

BRAHMI

Has traditionally been used for nervous disorders, epilepsy, senility, premature aging, hair loss, and obstinate skin conditions; considered to be the primary Ayurvedic nerve and cardiac tonic; also available in oil form.

CHANDRAPRABHA

Not a single herb, but rather a traditional formula used to maintain healthy cholesterol levels and blood sugar levels, while supporting proper weight control; also useful for those prone to frequent urination.

CHYAVANPRASH

A famous herbal jam made from amalaki fruit; fortified with over 20 herbs to rejuvenate and strengthen the immune system; one of the highest sources of vitamin C.

GINGER

Beneficial for reducing nausea; ginger root may also inhibit the production of prostaglandins and leukotrienes which may contribute to pain and inflammation.

GOKSHURA

A rejuvenating herb used in Ayurveda to support proper function of the urinary tract and prostate.

GUDUCHI

Considered a bitter tonic and powerful immunomodulator; regarded as a blood purifier and liver protector; also considered helpful in eye disorders, and for promoting mental clarity.

GUGGUL (GUGGULU)

A gum resin, historically used for its antiseptic and deep penetrating actions in the treatment of elevated blood cholesterol and arthritis; often used as a carrier and combined with other herbs to treat specific conditions.

GYMNEMA

Commonly referred to as "Gurmar, the destroyer of sugar;" traditionally used in formulas to control blood sugar levels in the body.

HARITAKI

Used for coughs, asthma, abdominal distention, tumors, and itching; one of three herbs used in triphala, the primary Ayurvedic tonic for maintaining health.

KUTKI

A bitter and pungent herb used by Ayurvedic practitioners to support proper function of the liver and spleen.

HOLY BASIL

Offers a wide range of health benefits, principally supporting the respiratory system.

MANJISTA

Considered to be one of the best blood purifying herbs in Ayurveda; said to cool and detoxify the blood, dissolve obstructions in blood flow, and clear stagnant blood from the system.

NEEM

Considered to be one of the best healing and disinfecting agents for skin diseases and an anti-inflammatory for joint and muscle pain; also available in oil form.

SHATAVARI

Traditionally used to help stomach ulcers, inflammation and chronic fevers, and to provide support for the female organs.

TURMERIC

An herb in the ginger family used as a medicine, and used abundantly for color and flavor in Indian cuisine; believed to strengthen overall body energy, relieve gas, dispel worms, improve digestion, and dissolve gallstones; considered useful for relieving arthritis pain because of its anti-inflammatory properties; when taken internally, along with cayenne pepper, in an animal study, it significantly lowered inflammation.

Chinese herbs

The knowledge of using herbs for their healing properties has been passed down through the centuries in China. Generally speaking, Chinese herbs are safer than most western pharmaceuticals and rarely have unpleasant side effects.

When prescribed by a professional, Chinese herbs are usually able to eliminate or substantially reduce the symptoms of discomforts such as nausea, insomnia or headaches in a relatively short time, but healing of more intense illnesses may take much longer. That's because herbs are a form of food, so their effect on the body is very subtle. They provide a form of nutritional support so that the body is better able to respond to its own natural healing abilities.

The therapeutic qualities of each herb are dependent on how it's cultivated, harvested, and stored. Herbs must then be selected for their quality, and processed in the most effective way to increase their potency.

Herbs can be processed in several ways. They can be prepared as a tea (decoction) to draw out their medicinal qualities, or they can be sliced to increase their surface area and potency. Another method uses alcohol to extract the volatile oils.

You'll often see the purpose of each herb described as being warming, cooling, tonifying or purging. That's in keeping with the fact that Chinese herbalists use the eight principles of Chinese medicine to evaluate the symptoms that need to be treated. These are the same principles used in acupressure—internal/external, cold/hot, deficient/excess, yin/yang.

It's very important to use the correct herb, or the correct variety of an herb, to achieve the desired benefit. Ginseng, an herb that's used to support energy or Chi (Qi), is a good example of this. It comes in several different types, and the quality may also vary. If a particular variety is helpful for an individual who is weak, energetically cold, or generally deficient, this same variety could actually have undesirable effects if it is given to someone who is energetically warm. This illustrates why it can be very important to seek professional guidance when you're making herbal choices for your pet.

Combining herbs may make them even more effective because certain herbs used together may have a more potent synergistic effect than using either herb by itself. Since this is the case, anyone who would like to try using multiple Chinese herbs, especially to relieve symptoms of a chronic illness, should consult a trained herbalist who is knowledgeable and experienced in the proper combining of such herbs, or, at the very least, use a professionally prepared herbal formula.

Here's a list of just a few of the many Chinese herbs you may find helpful in treating yourself or your pets:

ALMOND KERNEL (xing ren)

Bitter, warm, slightly poisonous; moistens and lubricates the intestines and can promote regular bowel movements; used for all kinds of coughs, especially coughs from a cold.

ASTRAGALUS (huang qi)

Sweet, slightly warm; strengthens vitality, stamina, resistance to disease; improves adrenal gland, liver and digestive function; useful for treating bladder infections and preventing the formation of kidney stones; improves the ability to cope with physical and emotional stress.

BAD HE (filly bulbs)

Sweet, slightly bitter, slightly cold; moistens the lungs, clears heat, and alleviates coughs and sore throats; clears the heart and calms the spirit; used for insomnia, restlessness and irritability, especially in an illness accompanied by fever.

BEI CHAU HU

Long history of use in a variety of conditions, including liver disease and allergies; also used as a sedative; it's anti-inflammatory effect helps with arthritis.

BLACK SESAME SEEDS (hu ma ren)

Sweet, neutral; nourishes and fortifies the liver and kidneys, moistens and lubricates the intestines, and nourishes the blood; aids in recovery from fever, headache, numbness and dizziness caused by deficient blood or yin; relieves constipation and promotes regular bowel movements

CARDAMON (bai dou kou)

Pungent, warm, and aromatic; transforms dampness, warms the middle burner (the spleen and digestive system), moves Qi and transforms stagnation.

CODONOPSIS (clang sheng)

Sweet, neutral; tonifies the middle burner and benefits Qi; tonifies lungs, nourishes fluids, helps with chronic fatigue; has been used for centuries to treat appetite loss, diarrhea and vomiting; shown in animal studies to prevent the formation of peptic ulcers brought on by stress.

DA ZAO (black dates) or HONG ZAO (red dates)

Sweet, neutral; tonifies the spleen, benefits the stomach, nourishes Qi, moistens dryness, calms the spirit and harmonizes the harsh characteristics of other herbs. The black dates have a smoky flavor, and neither variety is as sweet as other types of dates in common use.

DIOSCOREA (shun yao)

Wild yam root; sweet, neutral; benefits both the yin and yang of the lungs and kidneys; tonifies the spleen and stomach; can be used powdered or cut up into pieces.

FRESH GINGER (sheng)

Disburses cold, warms the middle burner, adjusts and nutures protective Qi.

FOX NUT (qian shi)

Sweet, astringent, neutral; strengthens the spleen, stabilizes the kidneys; used for deficient kidney Qi patterns.

GOTU KOLA

A traditional herb of both Chinese and Ayurvedic medicine; has antioxidant activity that protects the body from damage by free radicals; is particularly useful for stress-related disorders and memory problems.

JOBS TEARS (yi yi ren)

Sweet, bland, cool; promotes urination, leaches out dampness, clears damp heat, used for edema; has a mild effect on deficient spleen patterns.

LONGAN FRUIT (long yan rou)

Sweet, warm; tonifies the heart and spleen; nourishes the blood and calms the spirit.

LOTUS SEEDS (lian zi)

Sweet, astringent, neutral; clears heartfire, nourishes the kidneys and strengthens the spleen; used in deficient patterns.

LYCII BERRIES (you qi zi)

Sweet, neutral; nourishes and tonifies the liver and kidneys; used for deficient blood and yin patterns with symptoms such as sore back and legs; could be beneficial for diabetics.

MUSHROOMS (Maitake, Reishi, Cordyceps)

Among the most powerful immune-supporting substances in the world; need to be of the organically grown variety to avoid the possibility of being contaminated by toxic substances in the ground in which they're grown.

PORIA COCOS (fu ring)

Sweet, bland, neutral; leaches out dampness of the middle burner (the spleen and digestive system); quiets the heart and calms the spirit.

SCHISANDRA

Astringent, soothing; a highly regarded Chinese herb; gradually corrects imbalances and brings the body's systems into equilibrium; useful as a kidney tonic, for diarrhea therapy, and especially for the respiratory system; used for race horses and polo horses as an endurance tonic to increase their stamina and help them quickly recover from exertion; also appropriate for working dogs.

ZIZIPHUS JUJUBA (suan zao ren)

Sweet, sour, neutral; nourishes the heart and liver and calms the spirit; used to treat irritability, insomnia and anxiety brought about by deficient blood or yin; can facilitate significant weight reduction according to some studies; should be used in the form of a very fine powder.

* * *

Now that you're aware of some of the many helpful herbs which are available, you'll need to know what form of herbal remedy to use, and how to administer whatever form you choose. In the next two chapters, we'll explore a variety of methods that will make this process easier for your pet.

Chapter 12

How to Administer Herbs - Part I

Capsules, tablets, powders, liquids

As a general rule, you can administer herbs in whatever way is easiest for you and most acceptable to your pet.

Herbs are available in many forms. You can grow fresh herbs in your own garden or even in small pots in your kitchen window. Some can also be harvested if you're able to find them growing wild in areas that are free from pesticides. Many fresh herbs are also available in supermarkets and some health food stores. Other herbs are already dried or powdered, and still others, especially those for medicinal use, come in capsule, tablet or liquid (tincture) form. When you're selecting fresh or dried herbs, be sure to choose those with good color and a pungent scent.

Here are some helpful guidelines for administering herbal remedies to your pets:

- Herbs usually work best if they're taken *away* from meal times. That's because all of the beneficial properties are better absorbed when the herb doesn't have to compete with a whole meal.
- Some herbs, like Boswellia, however, have properties that make it important to take them with adequate food. One source even recommends that you always dilute *liquid* herbs by mixing them into some food and hand feeding that amount. Or the herbs can be mixed with slippery elm powder and some filtered water and then given orally or in food.
- If the herb comes in a *powdered form,* you will need to mix it in with just a little bit of food.
- Herbs which have a bitter taste will definitely need to be mixed in with a small quantity of food to disguise the bitterness so your pet will take them.

- If the herb comes in a *capsule*, you can open the capsule and mix the contents in with a small amount of food, or wrap a little moist food around the capsule and serve it as a treat.

- Herbs that come in *tablet* form can also be hidden in a little moist pet food and served as if they're a special delicacy. Peanut butter, cheese, liver and sardines may also work well for this purpose.

- If you need another method to make swallowing a *tablet* easier, coat it with a little virgin coconut oil, olive oil, or even butter if necessary, to disguise the herbal taste and make the tablet slide right down. Sometimes when a pet isn't feeling well, we simply need to use anything that works in order to entice them to take the herbs or medications they need.

- *Tablets* can also be crushed and put in with just a little food when you need to give them to smaller animals.

- Herbs that come in *liquid* form (tinctures) can be put directly into a pet's mouth. However, tinctures should be diluted first, since pets usually don't like the taste of the alcohol. For dogs, 4-8 drops twice a day should suffice.

- To give *drops* to a dog, keep the dog's nose level or slightly pointed downward. Create a pouch between the lower teeth and the cheek. Quickly squirt the *drops* into the pouch and hold the mouth closed. To get the dog to swallow, stroke his neck or blow lightly on his nose. Don't pull up on the dog's head or try to tilt it backwards. In this position, the liquid could go down the windpipe instead of the throat. For a detailed description about how to administer both pills and liquids to dogs, you'll find more information, including photographs, at these two websites: *www.vetmed.wsu.edu:80/clientED/dog_meds.asp.*
  www.dummies.com/WileyCDA/DummiesArticle/id-688,subcat-PETS.html

- To give *drops* to a cat, gently grasp the sides of his cheeks with your left thumb and forefinger. Tilt his head back just enough to make his mouth open slightly. Hold his head securely and put the tip of the dropper into the side of his mouth. Squeeze out about half of the liquid. When he stops smacking and swallowing repeat these steps until you've administered all of the liquid from the dropper. Don't try to put the drops far back in the throat because this could cause choking or vomiting. You'll find more

information about administering liquids to cats at this website:
http://cats.about.com/cs/catmanagement101/ht/giveliquidmeds.htm

- If an herb comes in *fresh* form, it may need to be pulverized or converted into a powder first so that it can then be added to a little food. This can be accomplished by bruising, grinding or mashing. Bruising is done by placing the root on a hard surface and hitting it with a mallet. A leafy malleable herb can be bruised very quickly. Some parts of herbs may be mashed using a mortar and pestle, and some of the harder, thicker parts may even need to be ground up in a blender or coffee grinder.

- Some herbs can be made into *teas* for drinking or for external applications. The next two chapters will provide detailed information about herbal teas and compresses.

- If you think your pet needs to take multiple herbs at the same time, it may be a wise idea to consult an experienced herbologist or use a professionally prepared product which is already blended using the appropriate combination of herbs.

- Since certain herbs may cause slight nausea when taken on an empty stomach, if you see any signs of upset, then always feed those herbs with a small amount of food, or give them right after a full meal.

- If your pet definitely develops an upset stomach, stop using that particular herb. Many times that single dose may be all that was necessary to help the body begin to do the job it has now been activated to do.

- When symptoms seem to get worse instead of better right after using a remedy, this is sometimes called a "healing crisis." It's actually a sign that the remedy is working. Toxins are being pulled out of the cells so they can be eliminated from the body. Improvement usually follows a worsening of symptoms once the body has eliminated those toxins.

- If your pet seems to have a reaction to an herbal remedy, you can then try using the herb again in a smaller amount once those uncomfortable effects have passed. However, if your pet's condition doesn't improve, you need to seek professional advice.

- It's always wise to start your pet on the lowest dose possible and work your way up to a higher dose if it's needed.

- Herbs resonate with the body so it's not always necessary to increase the amount of an herb to get a better result. You may just need to use the herbs for a long enough time.
- Some herbal remedies are sold primarily for human consumption but are also safe for pets, and are used by veterinarians. There are no precise dosages for animals but, generally speaking, if a human takes a whole capsule (based on a human weight of 150 lbs), then feed a small pet a quarter of that amount and a medium to large pet, half of the dosage. Better yet, there are also herbal products which are designed specifically for pets. You can easily find an abundance of them on the internet by doing a search on herbs+pets, herbs+dogs or herbs+cats.

* * *

The two tables that follow are *suggested dosage guidelines* for using herbs for general nutritional support. You'll need to decide what the best amount is for your own pet. Remember to start with the lowest reasonable amount.

Weight	Liquid	Size 00 Capsule	Tea
5-10 lbs	2 drops	½ capsule	1 tsp
10-20 lbs.	4 drops	1 capsule	2 tsp
20-30 lbs.	6 drops	1 capsule	1 tbsp
30-50 lbs.	6-10 drops	2 capsules	4 tsp
50-70 lbs.	10-14 drops	2capsules	5 tsp
70-90 lbs.	14-18 drops	2 capsules	2 tbsp
90-110 lbs.	18-22 drops	4 capsules	3 tbsp

Liquid Dosage – Animals by size	
Toy dog/cat	3-5 drops mixed in meals, 3x daily
Medium dog	25 drops mixed in meals, 3x daily
Medium/large dog	40 drops mixed in meals, 3x daily
Horse	100 drops added to carrot or food, 3x daily

* * *

You now have at your fingertips a variety of methods for helping your pets by using herbal remedies, yet it's unwise to assume that herbs alone can restore the health of your pets. While herbs alone may relieve minor problems, most holistic veterinarians recommend nutritional support, plus conventional therapy, plus herbs if the problem is acute, severe or life threatening. This integrated approach is designed to give the animal the greatest amount of comfort, combined with the gentlest and most effective treatments.

Before using herbal remedies for your pet, it's also important to do your own research. There's a wealth of information available, both on websites and in books. But just as you're doing with the material I've provided, consider most of what you read only as a suggestion or guideline. For expert advice, find an experienced veterinary herbalist in your area who can give you the professional guidance you need for your own pet. I know I repeat this caution every so often, but that's because it's so important.

Next, we'll explore the use of a wide variety of techniques for using herbs in various forms including teas, tinctures, elixirs, compresses, poultices and packs.

Chapter 13

How to Administer Herbs—Part 2

Herbal tinctures, elixirs, teas, rinses, compresses, poultices and packs

Herbal tinctures, elixirs and teas are some of the best ways to administer herbal remedies internally because they're all in liquid form, and therefore more fully and quickly absorbed by the body. The herbal fluids reach the blood stream much faster than they do when herbs are used in other forms because they're directly absorbed through the tissues of the mouth.

While powders, capsules and tablets can be very useful forms for administering herbs, they're usually a little less potent because they have to travel all the way through the stomach and digestive system first, and they may lose some of their effectiveness in that process.

In addition to giving herbal formulations to your pet internally, there are times when you need to relieve your pet's discomfort externally as well. Herbal rinses, compresses, poultices and packs are all very effective methods you can use for this purpose. They provide a unique type of herbal support for your pet's body during the healing process.

In the previous chapter, we discussed how to administer herbal powders, capsules and tablets to pets. In this chapter, we'll look in detail at each of the other forms of administering herbal remedies.

Tinctures

A tincture is a liquid extract, usually preserved with alcohol or vegetable glycerin. It's a very concentrated form of an herb which is easy to administer.

Alcohol is the most widely used tincture preservative because it keeps the solution fresh and stable for a longer period of time. However, for a pet with liver problems, you may prefer using a tincture preserved with vegetable glycerin. This is called a glycerite compound.

Adult dogs and cats may safely take tinctures, but they're not recommended for puppies, kittens, birds, rabbits and other small creatures.

Tinctures are only to be taken internally. Because of the alcohol preservative, they're not meant to be used full strength for external application, although if they're diluted with a sufficient amount of water, they may be used to moisten a compress, as you'll read about later in that section.

Tinctures have a very strong taste and some animals may object to it. If so, you can always dilute the tincture with water, or, if necessary, a little no-sodium or low-sodium broth. If tinctures don't work for your pet, try using an elixir (described below) instead.

Many tinctures are available in prepared form, but here are the directions for making your own if you need to do so.

- Put ½ cup dried or 1 cup fresh chopped herb into a dark colored glass jar with a tight cover.
- Add 2 cups of brandy or vodka that is more than 60 proof.
- Put the glass jar in a warm, dark place and shake it twice daily for 2 weeks.
- Strain through double muslin, squeezing the herb.
- Store the tincture in a covered, dark-colored glass jar. This preparation will last for several years.
- Put a small quantity into a separate dark-colored bottle for regular use. This will help the rest of the tincture remain fresher for a longer period of time because it won't be so frequently exposed to air.
- Use only as many drops as necessary each time. Dosage for adult dogs up to 50 lbs is 2 to 4 drops. For dogs up to 125 lbs, use 4 to 8 drops. Dosage for adult cats is 1 to 2 drops.

Elixirs

An elixir is a tincture which has been diluted with a sufficient amount of water. This maintains the therapeutic effect, but it decreases the strong flavor. Elixirs are meant to be taken only internally.

To make an elixir from an herbal tincture:

- Put 3 drops of herbal tincture into a one ounce bottle that has a glass dropper.
- Fill the dropper bottle 2/3 full with cool or room temperature distilled water.
- Cover and shake vigorously 108 times.

- Shake 12 times before each use.
- Dosage is ¼ dropper given a full 20 minutes before meals or treats. Most full droppers contain 20 drops, so ¼ dropper should yield about 5 drops.
- Keeps in refrigerator for up to 7 days.

Because elixirs are already a mixture that's been diluted with water, they're usually safe for all animals to use.

Teas

A very effective way to use herbs for healing purposes is to make a tea with them. Teas can be used internally, and they can also be used to make rinses and compresses for external applications. You'll find specific directions for several ways to use herbal teas for your pets as you continue reading.

When most of us talk about making tea, we usually think only about boiling some water and dropping a tea bag or some fresh herbs into it, but there are actually several interesting and effective ways to prepare herbal teas.

Infusion

An infusion is a simple form of hot tea made with boiling water. This is what you might call an every-day form of making tea.

Teas can be made with either the dried or fresh herb, using a single herb or a combination of herbs. You may choose to use the flower, the stem, the root, the seed, the leaves and/or the fruit. Always use organically grown herbs whenever possible.

- Start by boiling spring or distilled water.
- In an appropriate heatproof container, put 1-2 teaspoons of dried herbs, or 3-4 teaspoons of fresh herbs. Add about 12 ounces of boiling water.
- Let stand (or *infuse*), covered, for 10-15 minutes for most herbs. Black teas require less steeping time, while white and green teas require considerably more steeping time to bring out their flavors.
- If you're using other forms of herbs, it's recommended you use tea leaves and not pre-packaged tea. The leaves will fall to the bottom during the infusion time.
- Strain the preparation, and use it when it reaches a comfortable temperature for drinking. Any remaining tea may be refrigerated for up to 48 hours if necessary.

Cold infusion

A cold infusion is a method of preparing a tea without using boiling water.

- Soak 6 teaspoons bruised fresh herb or 2 teaspoons dried herb in about 12 ounces of cool water for 8 to 12 hours. (Bruising is the act of placing the herb on a wide, thick board and smashing it with a wooden mallet.)
- Strain and use. Refrigerate the remaining portion.

Decoction

A decoction is a simmered or boiled tea using roots, bark, stems, or seeds.

- Put 1 ounce bruised or crushed herb into a small saucepan with 2 cups of cool or room temperature distilled or spring water.
- Bring to a boil and let simmer for 30 minutes. The water should be half gone by the end of that time, but if more than half has evaporated sooner than that, then you'll need to add some additional water before the end of the simmering time.
- Turn off the heat and let the decoction stand covered until cool.
- Strain and use, or refrigerate if necessary for up to three days.

Storing herbal teas

Air, light, moisture, and odors from other foods can all reduce the amount of time that tea can retain its freshness.

While all of the directions above suggest refrigerating the leftover tea, another source recommends against refrigerating or freezing tea at all. It suggests instead, that leftover tea should be stored in a cool dry place in a container that is airtight and won't let light in (no clear glass containers).

Administering herbal teas to pets

If your pet will freely drink herbal tea from a bowl, you can serve it to him that way. When you feel he's had a sufficient amount, simply remove the bowl until the next day. Pets usually know when they've had enough, so they're not likely to drink too much of it.

If, however, you need to give the tea along with food, don't put the whole dose of tea in with all of the food for an entire meal. If your pet doesn't like the taste, he may decide to skip that meal altogether. Instead, to mask the taste and be sure he receives a complete dose, mix the tea in with just a little bit of food and serve this smaller quantity two or three times each day. If your pet is hesitant to eat one of these small servings, you may then need to be creative and add other tempting morsels to the food/tea mixture to further help mask any undesirable taste.

Dosages

Suggested dosages would be 1 tablespoon of herbal tea per 25 pounds of body weight. Based on that dosage, a 25 lb dog would receive a whole tablespoon and a 10 pound cat would be given about a ½ tablespoon. A bird would receive 1 ml per kilogram of body weight on a piece of cracker.

Herbal teas aren't as strong as herbal extracts or tinctures, so you may need to add a larger quantity of herbal tea to a meal, or coax your pet to drink a sufficient amount during the day, in order to achieve the same effect you would if you were using one of the more concentrated forms like a tincture or an elixir.

Speed of Action

How long does it take for an herbal tea to work? It could take up to 2 hours before it first takes effect. Long-range, a good rule of thumb when giving any herbal remedy to your pet is to use it for two weeks and than take one week off. That gives the body time to work on its own, and it gives you time to determine if the herbal treatment needs to be continued.

Rinses

A number of herbal teas are also very helpful to use as rinses. For example, green tea may be helpful for allergies, and a calendula rinse applied to the body can be soothing, healing and antimicrobial. It can be used on the skin, or even to soothe inflamed gums. If your dog has a sore throat or a bacterial infection in the upper gastrointestinal tract, put a cup of calendula tea in a quart of your pet's drinking water to help soothe those irritations.

To prepare a tea for a calendula rinse:
- Bring one quart of fresh water to a boil
- Add ½ cup of fresh dried flowers
- Simmer for 5-10 minutes
- Remove from heat, cover, and let steep until cool
- Strain, and freely apply the liquid infusion to skin irritations

To prepare a green tea rinse:
- Bring one quart of fresh water to a boil
- Add ½ cup of green tea if using loose leaves, or use 4 tea bags

- Simmer for 5 minutes
- Remove from heat, cover, and let steep until it reaches room temperature
- Strain if necessary, and freely apply the liquid to the affected areas on the skin

How effective are herbal tea rinses?

One of my clients has given me permission to share her successful experience with you. I recommended the use of Green Tea rinses to Rosandra awhile ago when her long-haired Chihuahua, Mika, was suffering from severe allergies. Since I wasn't going to meet Mika and her sister, Puddy, in person, Rosandra sent pictures of them before our phone consultation. My heart fell when I saw Mika's picture. She had red spots all over her face, her fur had fallen out in many places, and her left eye was swollen to the point of barely being open.

When we finally talked, Rosandra told me this was the way Mika usually looked. Several veterinarians and two specialists hadn't yet been able to determine the cause of her allergies. At the end of our consultation, I suggested to Rosandra that she try using a cold green tea herbal infusion to see if that would help minimize the swelling and relieve Mika's itchy skin. I also explained the basics of a raw food diet to her.

This is an excerpt from an e-mail I received from Rosandra just a few days later:

Dear Dr. Monica:

. . . Mika was a little better the rest of the weekend. We made some green tea, and after it cooled, I washed her little face with it. She didn't really want to let us do that, but by the time we finished with her face, she was putting her front paws into the tea, and she even started drinking some tea, too! I wasn't sure she should be drinking tea, but I thought it might help to sooth her.

Mika rested for a long time afterwards, without her Elizabethan collar. Her eyes didn't water as much, and the redness faded. It wasn't a cure, but it was a welcome relief. I'd like to continue using the tea infusions for Mika. They seem to be helpful for her.

We've also decided to stop using regular dog food to see if the itchiness clears up. We gave Mika a dinner based on the nutritional formula you gave us. Mika ate chicken, brown rice, and mixed veggies. Puddy decided she wanted to have some too. . .

Thank you for helping us. I will certainly be in touch,

Rosandra.

Several months later, Rosandra sent me this update:

Hello Dr. Monica,

. . . I wanted to let you know that since our session in January, Puddy and Mika are doing very well. You may recall that Mika had lots of allergies and you suggested changing her diet and steeping some tea to use to wash her face and the area around her eyes.

Mika has now come full circle! She enjoys a raw food diet and her allergies are down to a minimum. She has the occasional flare-up, but certainly not to the degree she did when you last saw her picture. Thank you for helping us get her on the right path. . .

Rosandra

From Rosandra's experience with Mika, it's easy to see how beneficial it can be for our pets to use healing herbal remedies like cold infusion tea rinses, along with a natural whole food diet.

Compresses

Compresses can be made with herbal teas by soaking a cotton or flannel cloth in a strong herbal tea solution, and applying the cloth to the affected area of the body.

To prepare a compress, dip the cloth into the herbal tea solution. Squeeze out the excess so the cloth is very wet but not dripping, then fold it into the appropriate size, and place it on the affected area for about 10 - 15 minutes.

Instead of using an herbal tea, you can also make a compress by soaking a cloth in a solution made up of 2½ tablespoons of tincture in 2 cups of hot or cold water.

It's helpful to use hot compresses when you need to increase circulation to some area of the body and you want the herbal properties to penetrate beneath the skin.

Heat also stimulates the absorption of cellular debris while an injury is healing and can help relieve neuralgia, boils, abscesses and cystitis. Hot, moist heat also relaxes contractions for whelping animals.

Probably the most popular use for a hot compress is to relieve the discomfort of muscular aches and pains caused by sprains or rheumatism, but heat should normally be used only after any inflammation has already subsided (24-72 hours).

In all of these cases, the compress must be very warm to be effective, but not so hot that it will burn. To maintain an effective level of warmth, have a second cloth available and alternate the cloths before the current one cools too much. If you have only one cloth available, re-heat it by dipping it into the hot tea several times during the application time.

Could you use dry heat instead? This is not recommended. Moist hot compresses are preferable to dry sources of heat like heating pads because dry heat may dehydrate muscles making them less flexible and predispose them to further injury.

Other circumstances will require the use of cold compresses, for example, when you need to ease skin rashes like eczema and psoriasis. Cold compresses also relieve inflammation, headaches, fever, indigestion, sprains and bruises.

Poultices

A poultice is a moist herbal pack which is applied directly to an external part of the body. The herbs in a poultice not only nourish the skin, but they can be absorbed into the lymph and blood vessels beneath the surface of the skin.

The properly prepared fresh or dried herbs for a poultice are usually wrapped in gauze, muslin, cheesecloth, bandages, or even, in an emergency, plastic wrap. The wrapped poultice can be applied directly to an inflamed, irritated, swollen, infected or injured part of the body (except to open wounds as you'll see below).

Reasons to use poultices

A poultice can be used to relieve external skin irritations, or for drawing out any type of unwanted material from under the skin. Poultices are also an excellent way of softening and dispersing material that has become hardened, such as scar tissue.

A hot poultice increases heat and circulation, while a cold poultice decreases heat and inflammation.

For skin flare-ups and hot spots, it's beneficial to apply a warm poultice (or a warm moistened herbal tea bag) directly to the affected area. The tannic acids of the tea ooze onto the skin and have a soothing, itch-relieving effect. This type of poultice may give the same type of relief as using cortisone cream. When the pet licks the area afterwards, he or she will also ingest some of the herbal residue. And it's definitely preferable for a pet to ingest herbs instead of ingesting topical cortisone by licking it.

You can apply this type of poultice twice daily for three days. To maximize the treatment, you can then apply aloe vera gel directly to the spot to further speed the healing process.

Cautions when using poultices

- A hot poultice can hold in heat for a considerable amount of time, so whenever you're using a hot poultice, be sure to take extra care to see that it's warm enough to be beneficial, but not hot enough to burn the affected area.
- Poultices may be left in place for only a short time, or when held with a bandage, they may be left in place for longer periods of time, but they should be changed periodically.
- If you're using a commercially prepared poultice which contains medications or irritants that could cause blistering, be sure to ask your vet about them first.
- *Apply a poultice only after the area has been thoroughly cleansed.*
- *Do not reuse a poultice.* Have a second poultice ready to apply before you remove the current one.
- *Do not generally apply a poultice over an open wound.* This may slow the healing process or allow infection to set in.
- *Do not generally apply a poultice to an injury until after your pet has been examined by a vet.* The effects of a poultice may mask the symptoms before a vet has a chance to evaluate the injury.

Preparing and using a poultice

To make a poultice, it's best to use herbs in powdered, crushed or chopped form. Mix them with enough hot water to make a thick paste. If you don't have ground herbs, boil the leaves or roots for a few minutes, then drain them. You can also use an herbal tea bag if necessary.

Apply the paste in a layer about 1/4 inch thick on a piece of cloth (cotton, muslin, cheesecloth, bandage, etc.). The cloth should be large enough to cover the affected area completely. Then cover the cloth with a piece of plastic—even a clean grocery bag will work in a pinch. The plastic should extend beyond the cloth by several inches on all sides.

It's not unheard of to place an unwrapped herbal poultice directly on unbroken skin, and then cover it with plastic, but this is rarely done, it's not normally recommended, and it should never be applied to an open wound.

Hold the poultice in place with a strip of cloth, or an ace bandage, or by pinning the ends of the covering together. If you have to use tape, you'll need to use extra care when removing it from skin or fur. If your pet doesn't try to remove it, you can leave the poultice in place for up to an hour at a time.

Packs

Packs are another form of healing treatment. Here are suggestions for making two different types of packs:

Pack 1

Saturate a piece of flannel cloth with castor oil and apply the pack to an area of the body where there's congestion. The oil can be warmed first by placing it in a container and setting the container in a pan of hot water. The oil in these packs has a drawing power of about four inches within the body and can help alleviate many conditions including muscular tension, back pain and liver toxicity.

Pack 2

Grind up some fresh comfrey leaves and pour hot water over them. Then drain off the water leaving an herbal mush of softened leaves. Take the warm herbal mush and wrap it in a cloth. Hold the cloth against the affected area for ten minutes twice a day. This type of a pack is helpful to relieve inflammation and swelling, and can also be used after surgical stitches have been removed.

* * *

In the next chapter, you'll find recipes for a number of herbal teas to help ease a variety of your pet's discomforts.

Chapter 14

Herbal Tea Recipes

The following herbal tea recipes have been designed to relieve the pain and discomfort associated with a number of the more common problems your pets may experience. The source for some of these recipes is the book *The Last Chance Dog*, by Donna Kelleher, DVM.

It's best to prepare teas in a glass or stainless steel container. If you're using a teakettle or saucepan, please be sure it's not aluminum.

As you learned in the previous chapter, herbal teas can be taken internally or applied externally as a compress, and some can be used in both ways.

How long a tea should be used will depend on some of its ingredients or on the nature of the problem. There are no hard and fast rules, but plan on about two weeks for internal use and even up to a month for external use. If the herbs you're using don't seem to be working, it may then be time to try a different herb, or consult a professional.

Recipes which contain Oregon Grape Root or Goldenseal, however, should only be used for a limited amount of time. (See section on **Herbs To Be Used With Caution** in Chapter 10).

Dosages for dogs and cats are indicated below. For birds and other exotic pets, give 1 ml per kilogram of body weight on a cracker. For example, an average cockatoo would be given 0.5 ml twice a day.

Wound-healing tea

This tea can be used *externally* on all animals for hot spots, chronic abrasions, or wounds that won't heal.

Ingredients:

3 quarts bottled or purified water
1/3 cup cut plantain leaf
1/3 cup cut comfrey leaf
1/3 cup packed calendula flowers (fresh is best)
1/3 cup chamomile flowers

1/3 cup packed yarrow flowers
2 tablespoons aloe vera gel (fresh is best)
2 tablespoons powdered Oregon grape or goldenseal root

Directions:

Combine all of the ingredients in a large saucepan, cover, and simmer for 15 minutes. Remove from heat, uncover, and let cool.

Strain the tea and discard the solids. Keep the tea in the refrigerator where it will last for up to three weeks.

Apply to the skin either as an herbal compress or by using a cotton ball. Let the tea stay in contact with the skin for at least 5 minutes twice a day. Do not rinse with water afterwards. Leave the tea on the skin. As soon as the affected area improves, discontinue the applications. If the skin is red and inflamed, the tea should be allowed to cool before applying it.

Although all teas can be used for drinking, this tea is a fast acting combination of herbs that is better used externally.

Hot-spot and allergy herbal tea

This recipe helps to keep pets from licking or chewing on hot spots, on incisions after surgery, or on areas of redness caused by allergies.

Ingredients:

2 quarts fresh bottled or filtered water
½ cup calendula flowers
¼ cup chamomile flowers
¼ cup yarrow flowers
¼ cup comfrey leaves
¼ cup grindelia flowers
1/8 cup plantain leaves
2 tablespoons goldenseal powder

Directions:

Combine all of the ingredients in a saucepan and simmer over low heat for 10 minutes. Remove from heat and uncover. Let steep and cool for 2-3 hours. Then strain the tea and discard the solids.

Warm the tea to room temperature before each application. Apply the tea as a compress, or use a cotton ball on the affected area for 10 minutes, 2-4 times a day.

This tea will last up to three weeks in the refrigerator.

Respiratory support herbal tea

This tea is beneficial for pets with kennel cough, pneumonia, infectious bronchitis and sinusitis.

Ingredients:

1 ½ quarts low-sodium chicken broth or water

1/3 cup cut Echinacea leaves

¼ cup cut Oregon grape or goldenseal root or 2 tablespoons powdered herb

¼ cup cut marshmallow root

¼ cup cut mullein leaves

1/8 cup grated fresh ginger root

1/8 cup cut elecampane root

Directions:

Combine all ingredients in a saucepan and simmer over low heat for 20 minutes. Remove from heat and set the covered pan in a cool place for 6-10 hours. Strain the tea, and discard the solids.

The tea will last about 10 days in the refrigerator. You can freeze some of it into ice cubes and thaw as needed for use.

Always bring the amount of tea you're going to use to room temperature before administering. Give 1 tablespoon of tea per 25 lbs of a dog's weight. For cats, give ½ tablespoon twice daily. It can be given by syringe, or with a small amount of food, or drunk from a bowl. Use for 10-14 days.

Bronchial congestion herbal tea:

Ingredients:

Coltsfoot (Tussilago farfara)

Mullein (Verbascum thapsus)

Horehound (Marrubium vulgare)

Directions:

Place 1 tablespoonful of each herb in a large teapot. Fill the pot with boiling water and infuse the herbs for at least 10 minutes. Pour out half a teacupful through a strainer. Sweeten with honey if necessary to reduce the bitterness of the horehound.

Always bring the amount of tea you're going to use to room temperature before administering. Give 1 tablespoon of tea per 25 lbs of a dog's weight. For cats, give ½ tablespoon twice daily. It can be given by syringe, or with a small amount of food, or drunk from a bowl while the tea is warm. Use for 10-14 days.

Urinary tract infection herbal tea

Ingredients:

1 ½ quarts low-sodium chicken broth or water

1/3 cup cut yarrow flowers

¼ cup cut Oregon grape or goldenseal root or 2 tablespoons powdered herb

¼ cup cut plantain leaves

¼ cup Uva Ursi leaves

¼ cup cut corn silk or marshmallow root

Directions:

Combine all ingredients in a saucepan and simmer over low heat for 20 minutes. Remove from heat and set the covered pan in a cool place for 4-6 hours. Strain the tea and discard the solids.

The tea will last about ten days in the refrigerator. You can freeze some of it into ice cubes and thaw as needed for use.

Always bring tea to room temperature before using. Give 1 tablespoon of tea per 25 lbs of a dog's weight. For cats, give ½ tablespoon twice daily. It can be given by syringe or with a small amount of food, or drunk from a bowl. Use for 10 to14 days.

Muscle spasm herbal tea

This tea is beneficial for muscle spasms and it also helps to reduce inflammation and pain.

- Crampbark helps relax muscles.
- Corydalis root has been used for centuries for pain, and contains an ingredient similar to morphine, but much less potent.
- Meadowsweet is an original source of aspirin or salicylic acid.
- Boneset is a tonic and mild laxative.

Ingredients:

4 cups water or low-sodium chicken broth

¼ cup crampbark

¼ cup corydalis root

¼ cup meadowsweet leaves

1/8 cup boneset

Directions:

Combine all of the ingredients in a saucepan, cover and simmer over low heat for 30 minutes, trying to keep evaporation to a minimum. Turn off the heat and leave the pan covered for 4-6 hours. Strain the tea, and discard the solids.

Keep in the refrigerator but bring to room temperature before using.

Externally, this recipe can be used in a compress. Internally, give 1 tablespoon of tea per 25 lbs of a dog's weight until muscle spasms subside. For cats, give ½ tablespoon twice daily. It can be given either by syringe, or with a small amount of food, or drunk from a bowl.

Hypothyroidism herbal tea

Ingredients:

4 cups low-sodium chicken broth or water
2 whole roots red Chinese ginseng
¼ cup hawthorn berries
2 tablespoons ground cinnamon
2 tablespoons ground turmeric
2 tablespoons grated fresh ginger root

Directions:

Combine all of the ingredients in a saucepan, cover and simmer over low heat for 20 minutes. Remove from the heat and set the covered pan in a cool place for 4 to 6 hours. Strain the tea, discarding the solids.

Give 1 tablespoon per 40 lbs. of a dog's body weight per day, in food, for the remainder of the pet's life. For cats, give about ½ tablespoon.

Imbalanced immune system herbal tea

This tea is good for either chronic of recurrent infections. It may be beneficial if your pet gets sick often or has enlarged lymph nodes. It's also helpful if laboratory test results show that your pet's white blood cell count is consistently very low and his globulins are high.

Ingredients:

1 ½ quarts low-sodium chicken broth or water
1 piece astragalus root, 2" x 8"
¼ cup cut rose hips
¼ cup cut pau d'arco bark
¼ cup cut alfalfa leaf

¼ cup cut gotu kola leaves
¼ cup cut cat's claw bark
2 tablespoons chlorella powder

Directions:

Combine all ingredients in a saucepan and simmer over low heat for 20 minutes. Remove from heat and set the covered pan in a cool place for 4-6 hours. Strain the tea and discard the solids.

This tea will last about 10 days in the refrigerator. You can freeze some of it into ice cubes and thaw as needed for use.

Always bring tea to room temperature before using. Give 1 tablespoon of tea per 25 lbs of a dog's body weight. For cats, give ½ tablespoon twice daily. It can be given by syringe or with a small amount of food, or drunk from a bowl. Use for 10-14 days.

Liver treatment herbal tea

This tea uses herbs which cleanse and support the liver.

- Dandelion leaves can help the liver clear out chemical toxins.
- Oregon grape root contains the yellow compound berberine, a natural antibiotic similar to goldenseal.
- Bupleurum is especially helpful for strengthening the sinews.
- Baical Scullcap cleanses dirty liver cells.
- Bhumy amalaki heals drug-induced liver damage.
- Milk thistle has the ability to help the body rebuild individual liver cells.

Directions:

Mix ¼ cup of each herb in 3 quarts of distilled water. Let it simmer for 15 minutes. Strain the tea and let it cool to room temperature.

Give dogs one teaspoon per 20 lbs of body weight mixed with food or broth, twice a day. Give cats about 3 ml or about ½ teaspoon twice a day. Use for 10 to 14 days.

This tea is bitter and some animals don't like it for that reason. You might try adding a little honey or molasses to mask the bitter taste, as long as your pet doesn't have diabetes. Usually it takes several weeks to start seeing an improvement. Give this tea until symptoms subside.

Relaxation herbal tea

Try this tea for pets who suffer from various kinds of distress, especially during fireworks season or thunderstorms. It can also be used for dogs who have to travel a lot, and for cats before taking a trip to the veterinary clinic.

Ingredients:

2 quarts low-sodium chicken broth or water
1/3 cup passionflower
1/3 cup chamomile flowers
¼ cup cut oatstraw leaves and stems
¼ cup packed hops flowers
¼ cup skullcap leaves
1/3 cup lobelia leaves
1 tablespoon powdered kava kava

Directions:

Combine all of the ingredients in a saucepan and simmer over low heat for 10 minutes. Remove from heat, uncover, and allow to steep for 4-6 hours.

Give 1 tablespoon per 25 lbs of a dog's body weight, 2 or 3 times a day. It takes about 2 hours to take effect. For cats, give ½ teaspoon.

Chapter 15

Exercising Your Pets For Optimum Health

Today, we're creating a generation of pets who are becoming fat and physically unfit because we overfeed and under-exercise them. This excess of food and lack of physical activity allows their bodies to become soft and weak. Poor body condition makes it difficult for them to handle the normal demands of daily living, and even more difficult for them to resist or overcome many health challenges.

Pets are now developing some of the same debilitating conditions we used to find only in people. These include stress and anxiety disorders, cancer, diabetes, heart disease, strokes and osteoporosis—most of which were never seen in animals until only fairly recently.

The good news is that most of these diseases or conditions can be prevented, and some can even be overcome, if our pets are given a high quality diet *and* high quality exercise.

Although this book is primarily about nutritional health for your pets, it wouldn't be complete if we didn't also address their physical, mental and emotional well-being. In the next several chapters, we'll talk first about what happens when pets don't get enough exercise and mental stimulation. Then we'll explore some interesting and clever ways to provide both enjoyable physical activity and mental stimulation for your pets.

Life in the animal kingdom—wild and domestic

For animals in the wild today, physical activity is an integral part of daily living. When they aren't resting, every moment of their existence is dedicated to finding food or shelter, protecting their territory, playing, or engaging in fight or flight. They're usually slim, trim and physically fit. This was also true for our animals' ancestors. But today, a serious lack of physical activity is a fact of modern life for most of our pets.

While animals in the wild still have to hunt for their food and shelter, our pets simply walk up to their bowls and watch as their food miraculously appears. For some animals, the trip to the kitchen may even be their longest walk of the entire day! Not only does their food appear without any effort on their part, but they can also count on having the security of guaranteed shelter and at least the basic comforts of life without having to search for them.

Animals in the wild regularly socialize and play freely with other pack members, but many of our pets live in single animal households, and never have the enjoyment or physical benefit of another animal to play or chase around with.

Like animals in the wild, sometimes pets who live in multi-dog households do have to contend with occasional fights. Most of the time, though, they're able to live with the situation. However, some pets live in a constant state of stress when there's a bully in the household. Unlike animals in the wild, the stressed-out pets often aren't able to find a safe haven because true flight is not an option for them. But most household pets rarely, if ever, have to give either fight or flight any thought.

It's fairly obvious from this comparison that our household pets aren't going to experience the same health benefits of physical activity as their counterparts in the wild do, unless *we* find interesting ways to provide them with plenty of regular exercise.

The truth about inactivity, confinement and boredom

Some people believe that dogs will get plenty of exercise if only they spend sufficient time in a large enough yard. The truth is that most dogs get little or no exercise when they're outdoors if they're by themselves. They spend most of their time lying around waiting for their people to play with them.

Pets who are inside the house alone are also waiting for their people to make their lives more interesting. They don't have a job, they aren't walked on a regular basis, and when the family does come home, sometimes after being away for 10 hours or more, the humans are so tired they go to sleep without so much as a walk around the block or the toss of a ball or frisbee.

Many of my pet clients complain about this. After long hours of boredom, these animals still receive little or no attention from family members, or at least not enough to make any significant difference in their lives. They're almost like incarcerated animals in a zoo.

But it's not natural for animals to be confined or inactive. Animals in the wild are on the move almost all day long. Most of our domestic breeds also have the same need to be physically active, especially when they're young. Unfortunately, though, many rarely have the opportunity.

Even a whole house or a yard can be a confined space for an animal who never regularly gets to travel into any other territory. And when animals are placed in confined spaces for long periods of time, without appropriate mental and emotional stimulation, plus plenty of physical activity, they can become crazed and even dangerous.

When this happens, they begin venting their frustration on any object within reach. Often this results in the destruction of carpets, doors, drapes, blinds, window shutters, wood sidings, screens, or any kind of furniture they can chew on.

Sometimes they'll even take out their frustration on another animal or on a person. And if a pet doesn't have some object to vent this kind of frustration on, he may then begin to vent it on himself.

I've seen some pets who have begun to bite and chew on themselves all day long. The results of this kind of behavior may even require medical intervention, but the behavior itself won't stop until a pet begins to receive adequate mental and emotional stimulation, as well as plenty of physical exercise.

Is it necessary for them to live this way, or for us to simply learn to put up with the physical and behavioral problems which inactivity and confinement bring about in our pets?

Absolutely not! Most of them could easily be corrected with a combination of optimum nutrition and a regular program of physical exercise that's enjoyable for both people and their pets.

* * *

You've already learned in the first part of this book how to meet your pet's nutritional requirements, but you also need to be certain they receive all of the healthful benefits of stimulating exercise. You can do this by creating plenty of entertaining play for them. The next two chapters will provide you with many interesting ideas you can try.

Chapter 16

Exercise For Dogs

Just as animals in the wild travel extensively during their waking hours, almost all of our domesticated pets also need some form of traveling on foot each day.

A dog who has been inactive for a long time should begin an exercise program starting with a slow paced walk every day for about 10-15 minutes.

As your pet becomes accustomed to a daily walk, begin to increase the pace at which the two of you move, as well as the distance you cover together, before allowing your pet to stop and sniff. After about a month, most pets should be able to manage up to an hour of good physical exercise each day.

If your dog is already a regular walker, why not make those walks more interesting? Ask your pet to carry something like a ball, a toy, or a newspaper while he walks. Let him carry his leash or ask him to "walk" another less experienced dog by carrying that dog's leash in his mouth.

In the United States, you can even find specially designed backpacks which your dog can wear to give him a greater sense of purpose. You can fill the pockets of the backpack with any appropriate items, including water bottles for both of you. If the backpack has some weight in it, then your pet receives the benefit of an additional work out whenever he's carrying a load appropriate to his age, size, and state of wellbeing.

Ideally you should walk your dog once in the morning, especially if he stays home alone all day, and once again in the evening after you come home. The average amount of exercise a dog needs will depend on the size, age and nervous energy of your pet. Generally a small breed will do well with about 20 minutes each time, while a larger breed, a young dog, or a high strung animal, will need up to an hour each time.

Walking can graduate into running for most dogs. If you aren't able to run yourself, try riding a bicycle, or using roller blades, a skateboard, or some other type of "wheels." Or maybe one of your neighbors who runs regularly could take your dog out occasionally.

How much exercise is appropriate?

It's important to consider your dog's breed, age and the state of his health when you're deciding how much exercise is appropriate.

No dogs of any breed should be subjected to a really demanding training routine until after they've fully completed the growing stage. Their bones, joints and muscles need to be well developed first.

For many breeds, the growth stage is completed by the time they're between nine and twelve months of age. However, giant breeds, like Great Danes and Saint Bernards, are not mature enough until they're at least eighteen months old.

Too much intense or prolonged exercise during these early months of development, especially for giant or larger breeds, may subject a dog to the risk of injury or permanent damage to their bones and joints. This doesn't mean that your puppy shouldn't be allowed to enjoy himself, but you do need to use good judgment and take extra care during his or her developmental period.

Giant breed dogs, as well as some larger dogs, even when they're fully grown, still don't have the ability to withstand vigorous activity because of their weight. Their large size predisposes them to overheating in only a short time, and it takes longer for them to cool down. For this reason, you need to be particularly mindful of their needs during hot and humid weather.

Breeds who have pushed in faces, like Shih Tzus, Pugs, Bulldogs, Boston Terriers, Boxers and Mastiffs find it more difficult to breathe, even after only a little exertion. They'll enjoy a good walk at a moderate pace for a moderate distance, but long hikes are not in their best interests. Hot weather also affects their ability to breathe, so they'll do much better with cooler morning or evening walks.

Dogs who have long spines, short legs, and hips that often develop poorly shouldn't be allowed to do too much exercise either. Breeds like Dachshunds and Pekingese will do well with a short, brisk walk but need to stay away from hills and hiking because they don't have the capacity for prolonged exertion.

On the other hand, the hounds, spaniels, terriers, collies, retrievers, pit bulls, and sled breeds have tremendous stamina. These dogs were bred to work all day long and they have the endurance levels to enable them to do it. The Akita is noted for its physical prowess, and the sight hounds, like the

Greyhound and the Afghan Hound, were born to run. Although they do very well in a home environment, they're at their best in an open field.

Healthy adult German Shepherds and Rotterweilers are usually able to out-run all but the most physically fit humans. One of my clients "advertises" this capability by putting up a sign on his large property that reads: German Shepherd Guard Dog: He can make it to the fence in 2.9 seconds. *Can you?*

Unfortunately, a number of larger breeds are genetically prone to hip dysplasia, which may be further aggravated if the dogs are exercised too strenuously at too young an age. Symptoms of hip dysplasia can range from mild to severe.

You'll definitely need the advice of your veterinarian to determine how much exercise is appropriate if your pet has this problem. Milder forms of this condition will actually be helped by some exercise, while more severe cases will be able to tolerate much less, and the worst cases will probably not be able to endure any prolonged activity at all.

Your dog's coat is also another factor to take into consideration when you're considering the appropriate level of activity for him.

Dogs with very short or sparse hair don't tolerate heat or cold very well, and may even be uncomfortable in unusually bright sunlight. They'll benefit from using sunscreens rated at SPF35 or higher to protect their sensitive skin when they're outdoors.

At the other end of the spectrum, dogs with very thick fur will also be affected adversely if they're trying to engage in too much physical activity during hot and humid weather.

Some people like to shave their long-haired dogs during the hot summer months, but this may have some unwanted consequences. Their skin is often very delicate so a short haircut will leave them less protected from the sun's rays, insect bites, fungal infections, and mite infestations. Simply shortening and thinning out their coats instead of shaving them may be the better part of wisdom.

When it comes to exercise, you're the one who must decide what's right for your pet at each different stage of his life. You don't want to injure him by forcing him to over-extend himself, so if your dog wants to stop, slow down, or turn back, let him do so!

This advice doesn't necessarily apply, though, to a dog who is just learning to exercise more vigorously. At first, a dog new to a program of high level physical activity may try to hold back because he's engaging in something he doesn't yet understand. For these pets, if they're young and healthy, and there's no apparent sign of any injury, be firm but loving as you teach them the ropes of physical fitness. Start with a short workout and only gradually increase the length and intensity.

A veterinarian, who's familiar with your dog's overall health and abilities, can always provide you with information and guidance when it comes to the appropriate level of exercise for your pet.

Some other exercise options

If the weather is not conducive to outdoor exercise, but your pet is healthy and walks well, then you can always put him on a treadmill if you have one.

If you do use a treadmill, *never ever leave your pet unattended for any reason whatsoever.* Accidents can happen in a flash, so you need to be present *at all times* to take immediate action if something should go wrong.

There are also many other entertaining ways to exercise your dog in addition to walking and running:

- Play a good 15-minute game of fetch or catch the frisbee.
- Play hide and seek by hiding something he likes and having him search for it.
- Take a long walk or run together at a local park.
- Provide supervised time in the swimming pool.
- If you have a yard, and your pet has a doggie friend in the neighborhood, schedule playtime together for the two of them.
- Take your pet to a dog park so he can socialize and play with other dogs.
- Let him spend one or more days each week at a doggie day care center.
- Enroll in an agility course where your pet will get plenty of exercise and be able to compete with other dogs.

Safety Tip: Whenever you're throwing the ball or frisbee, remember to throw it far, but not high. Jumping high into the air to capture it, but landing awkwardly, may lead to serious knee injuries.

Exercise safety tips

Whenever your dog is exercising, be sure to follow these tips:

- Safety first—always keep your dog on a lead whenever you walk or run. Even the best-trained dogs who are off leash can unexpectedly run into the path of a moving car. Using a leash is also a courtesy to other dog walkers, and is the law in many places.

- The more active your dog is, the more water he'll require. Make sure your pet has enough fresh water before and after your run. If the weather is very hot, or if you're going for a long run, always take some water along for both of you.
- Try to run on dirt paths or grass as much as possible. Things like gravel, concrete, hot asphalt, and road salt can irritate your pets paws.
- If you have to run when it's dark outside, put reflectors on your dog's collar, as well as on your own clothes.
- If it's freezing cold or hot and steamy out, keep your walk or run short, or play indoors instead.
- Keep a close eye on your pet when you're outside. Watch for any unusual signs of fatigue or difficulty breathing. If your pet wants to stop, then stop. Dogs who overdo it can suffer strained tendons or ligaments or other orthopedic problems. This is especially true for large and giant breed puppies when they're still growing.
- If your dog of any age regularly accompanies you, and one day simply stops in the middle of the road, always assume that he or she may have suffered some sort of injury like a muscle spasm, a cut foot pad, an accelerated heart rate, or a seizure. Never force a pet to continue physical activity until these conditions have been treated and fully healed.

Games to teach and play

If your dog likes treats, you can take advantage of his food interests to teach him some new games that will keep him active while entertaining him at the same time:

Tunnel exercise

Create a tunnel or a maze using some chairs or cardboard boxes. Encourage your dog to explore all the way to the other end by leaving some treats at the far end of the tunnel.

Concentration exercise

Hide some treats inside an old rolled-up towel. This is a lot of fun for your dog! The towel, however, may soon show some major signs of wear and tear!

Creative thinking exercise

Place a lightweight bowl face down over some hidden treats. A dog must use his creativity to turn the bowl right side up in order to find and eat all of the treats. This is another easy exercise—and fun for both you and your pet.

If your dog isn't that interested in treats, then try these two games:

Find it

Show your dog his favorite ball, toy, stuffed animal, or bone. Then, while he remains where he is on a stay command, go and place it in another room, out of his sight, but easily accessible. In the beginning, leave it in the middle of the room so that he can easily smell it and find it quickly. Repeat the words "Find it" or "Seek" while he's looking for it.

When he finds it and either looks at it, pounces on it, picks it up, or carries it off, then praise him enthusiastically. Make sure you play with him using whatever he's found before you hide it again.

As his skills improve, you can make the search more and more difficult by hiding the item in a more challenging place, or up higher than normal. This is an excellent exercise to do indoors when it's raining, snowing, or just too cold to go outside.

Retrieve it

It's always fun to teach a dog how to retrieve. Some dogs will go after the ball but won't pick it up and bring it back to you. Others will decide they'd rather play keep-away instead. For a dog who tries to take over the game, have a second ball handy and show him that as soon as he drops the first one, you'll throw the second one right away. Timing is everything. You need to practice consistently to help your dog master all of the steps in the art of retrieval—find it, pick it up, return it to you, and release it.

Most of all, have fun with your dogs. Remember, you're their pack leader and best friend, so they want to spend as much time with you as you can possibly spend with them.

Playtime safety tips

A couple of safety measures to observe whenever you're playing with your pets:

- Never use your hands or fingers as "bait," or as the object of teasing when you play with any animal. This teaches your pet that it's all right to bite and scratch not only your hands, but anybody else's hands, too. This kind of activity, while appearing to be fun, puts babies, children, visitors, or other adults in the home at risk.

- It's better not to let any pet chase a spot of light produced by a laser type flashlight commonly sold in pet stores nowadays. Some pet behaviorists say that this type of activity can trigger a state of severe obsessiveness in an animal which is very difficult to overcome, especially in certain dogs.

Give your dog a job

Dogs love to have jobs! One of the best things we can do for their wellbeing is to provide the mental stimulation that comes from having the responsibility of a specific task to perform regularly.

Those jobs may be as complex and physically demanding as herding other animals on a ranch, or as simple as responding to a command that requires mental concentration (and possibly the output of at least some physical energy) *every* time before they're given a meal or a treat. An animal who "works," and also receives excellent nutrition, will be a much healthier, happier pet.

While cats often find enough entertaining things to do on their own which satisfy their requirements for mental stimulation, most dogs will need to be given some activities that are much more structured. You can accomplish this by giving them a simple behavior to perform on command, or by giving them a more complex type of task to perform, one that may even require some very specialized training.

Some dogs have a highly developed sense of service, or have a natural ability to interact with people, or to herd other animals. We can often further develop and utilize these natural skills and abilities in very beneficial ways, while at the same time providing those animals with a challenging and satisfying job to do.

There are a wide variety of activities for dogs who respond well to specialized training. They can be Therapy Dogs, Service Dogs, Guide Dogs, and Hearing Dogs. They can be Search and Rescue Dogs, Detection Dogs, Police Dogs, Military Dogs, or dogs who otherwise guard and protect. In the Livestock industry, you'll find Herding Dogs and Livestock Guardian Dogs.

But not every animal is meant to perform such complex tasks, especially the kinds that require a high level of training.

Ranch and farm dogs engage in many different activities, often by themselves, or with only minimal training, but they're always on the alert, "thinking" about a variety of things they can do, and following through by taking appropriate action.

Then we have the typical household pets who lie around the house or yard much of the day, having no sense of any particular purpose in life and often feeling very bored. These are the dogs for whom we need to be the most creative when it comes to finding something they obviously enjoy doing, either to occupy themselves or to entertain us.

You can begin by giving your pet the "job" of performing standard behaviors like sit, sit up, down, roll (only half way), roll over, stand, and stay.

You can even "chain" some of these behaviors together, one after the other, while frequently alternating which one comes next, so that your pet never knows which command to expect from you.

At first, you can have your pet learn how to respond to verbal commands which are also accompanied by hand signals. Then later on, you can teach him to respond only to the silent hand signals alone. (Early training with silent hand signals can be especially helpful if your pet should ever lose his hearing later in life.)

Your unbridled enthusiasm when he performs each command successfully will do wonders to encourage him to continue because he'll feel he has something important to do, or that he's entertaining you. Praise is often all he'll require as a reward, though a food treat can also effectively be used, at least intermittently, especially when he's first learning new behaviors.

Next, you could progress to teaching tricks which require different levels of complexity and physical or mental activity. Your pet could learn to stand on his hind legs and dance, jump through a hula hoop, fetch his leash when it's time for a walk, bring in the newspaper, or come and find you to let you know when someone's at the door.

Once you've successfully taught these behaviors, be sure to let your dog "work" every day. Whenever he's using his skills to entertain you, other family members, or visitors, he'll feel a sense of importance and a responsibility to do his best, and you'll no doubt find you have a happier pet.

A word of caution . . .

Whenever you assign specific jobs you want your pets to perform, you need to clearly understand the importance *they* may attach to what they're being asked to do.

For example, I had a client who, every time she left home, would tell her Doberman that he was in charge of the house and yard and was supposed to protect them. While she was gone, he'd bark at anything that moved in the yard, and since they lived on a corner, he'd make sure every single person who walked by also knew he was in charge of guarding the property.

This client called to ask me for help because she was now very upset with him. Her dog was barking excessively when she was away from home, and her neighbors were now complaining about his behavior.

But he couldn't help it! He was just doing the job she'd given him to do!

When I talked to him, he was adamant that his mom was counting on him. He'd already scared off one possible intruder, and he was certain that if it hadn't been for him doing his job so well, the man would have gotten inside their home. This successful experience had doubled his enthusiasm for continuing to do his job effectively.

I fully explained the change in behavior that his mom now wanted to see, but nothing I told him ever convinced him to change the way he acted. He knew what she originally wanted, and he wasn't going to stop doing exactly what she'd requested, and what she'd reinforced over and over again for such a long time.

I finally had to tell his mom that it was going to be up to her to do everything she possibly could to change his perception of how she wanted him to behave whenever she was away from home. Never again should she tell him that she wanted him to guard the house and yard, or that he was in charge. He also needed something to do that would keep him well occupied, and above all, he needed plenty of very active physical exercise.

The last I knew about this big dog, who was so determined to do the job his mom had given him in the beginning, was that one day he mistook the woman's grandson for an intruder and went after him. She then felt the risk had become too great, and decided to give the dog away.

* * *

The moral of this story is: *Never tell your dog to do anything that puts him in a position of leadership.*

Most animals will instinctively defend their territory if no one else is home, but they should never be verbally encouraged to do so over and over again.

Instead, they should be given something interesting and safe to occupy their time alone. At other times, they should have a meaningful job to perform that doesn't put them in a position of leadership. And, above all, they should be given an abundance of exercise to help work off the stresses and frustrations that can build up from boredom.

Chapter 17

Exercise For Cats

And Other Animals

Cats are quite different from dogs when it comes to exercise. They're designed for short, frequent periods of intense activity, rather than for longer exercise sessions.

Just as different breeds of dogs require various levels of exercise, so do different breeds of cats. Activity that might be right for one, may not be right for another.

It's also important to keep in mind that cats are nocturnal animals so very often they're going to be more active after sundown. Some of my most mischievous clients are almost picture perfect all day long, but when night falls, they begin their loud screams and destructive behavior!

On the other hand, if your cat seems to sleep all the time, it's not necessarily a cause for concern. As long as cats are both physically and emotionally healthy, being quiet is perfectly normal for many of them. Some just enjoy being great lap cats who love to sit with you while you read or watch TV. It's even possible, if you're out of the house for many hours, that you're not seeing your cat at his or her most active times.

But every cat does need some exercise to maintain a healthy mind and body. If your cat isn't naturally active, then you need to entice her to play.

Some of the ways you can entice your cat into activity include giving her:

- **Things that can be hit.** Anything light weight that moves easily across the floor will give your cat a chance to practice hitting and chasing. Balled up tissue paper works well. Just make sure she's not batting anything she could chew up and swallow.
- **Things that can be chased.** The end of a moving string should bring out the predator in even the most sedentary cat. Again, just make sure your cat doesn't swallow the string. Mechanical animals can also be chased around the room.

- **Things that can be pounced on.** In the wild, cats hunt by slinking soundlessly and unseen through the brush, locating their prey, then pouncing. You can simulate this hunting experience by making a place where your cat can hide and then pounce, or by using a stick with some feathers on the end of it and moving it across the floor until she pounces on it and "catches her prey."
- **Things that can be climbed into.** Empty boxes and paper bags are perfect for this. Remember, plastic bags can cause suffocation, and lots of cats love plastic, so be careful.
- **Things that can be climbed on.** Tall "kitty trees" are wonderful because they let your pet climb almost to the ceiling which is something most of them love to do.
- **Things that can be scratched.** Scratching stretches and tones the muscles in your cat's shoulders and back as well as sharpening her nails. A scratching post—or even a piece of cardboard or carpet—can keep your pet active and keep your furniture safe. If your cat does scratch the furniture, try using double sided sticky tape on the sides of the sofa to deter her. Usually if her nails get "stuck" on a surface, she'll remember not to go there again!

Experiment with several types of toys. No matter which toy your cat likes best, remember that its appeal will increase if you'll put it out of sight in between play sessions.

To encourage stair climbing as exercise, if you have a multi-story home, place her food bowl on a different level from the one where she spends most of her time.

Some indoor cats can even be trained to walk outside on a leash. I have many clients who routinely do this. You need to start at a young age, though. The first step is letting your cat wear a harness inside the house for a few days so she can become used to the feel of it. Once she's comfortable with the harness, try attaching a leash and walking around inside the house together. Then walk around together in your own backyard if you have one. After that, using the harness and leash, you should be able to take walks outside together without worrying that your cat will run into the street, or run away.

You may even be able to allow your indoor cat to spend some time outdoors in an enclosed yard. However, her playtime outside may always need to be supervised, lest her natural instincts take over, prompting her to try to escape over the backyard fence.

If jumping the fence is a problem, you can find covered mesh "kitty runs" in some pet catalogs and on internet pet supply websites. These can be set up outdoors to allow your pet to enjoy spending some time closer to nature. She'll be able to move freely back and forth at ground level, and you won't have to be concerned that she might escape.

But in the end, if all of your efforts to engage your cat in more physical activity are met with a yawn, then maybe the best thing to do is simply accept her for who she is, pick up a book, and enjoy sitting beside her.

Exercise and other animals

Although we've only been talking about dogs and cats until now, keep in mind that almost all animals need exercise, regardless of their species or size.

Guinea pigs, mice, rats and hamsters are usually caged the majority of the time, but they do manage to get a fair amount of exercise when, or if, they're using running wheels.

Rabbits and birds, on the other hand, are often confined to cages most of their lives without being given much, if any, freedom to move around. Rabbits would definitely benefit from some daily exercise outside of their cages, and so would some types of birds. They both need a contained and secure environment, however, whenever they're allowed to be out of their normal habitats.

Horses often stand in their stalls for hours on end, or spend their time in small corrals. At the very least, they need to be walked every day, and allowed to run whenever possible to keep their muscles toned and their joints flexible.

Two species, reptiles and insects, are the exception to the rule about needing exercise. Both do well in confined spaces and generally don't take the opportunity to engage in physical activity, even if they're allowed or encouraged to do so.

But, if you have pets of any size, from a small mouse to a tall horse, make sure you give them plenty of daily exercise and loving human contact.

* * *

My hope is that you'll always remember: high quality nutrition plus high quality exercise provide the essential building blocks for optimum health for your pets. If you're successful in following many of the suggestions throughout this book, you should then have the companionship of healthy, happy, active pets for many enjoyable years.

Chapter 18

How to Pre-test Remedies

You're aware now of many helpful remedies which might be beneficial for your pet, but there may be times when you feel a little overwhelmed wondering which food, nutritional supplement or herbal remedy to select.

You've identified many items that may seemingly work well to treat your pet's specific symptoms or disease, but if you try too many different things at the same time, you have no way of knowing what's helpful and what's not.

It's also important to consider that some animals react well to a specific herb, nutritional supplement, food or medicine, while other animals with the same problem might react adversely. It's also valid to say that the same treatment or medicine might help an animal at one point during an illness, but not at another.

So how do you know which herb, nutritional supplement, food or treatment to use? Will your pet react positively or negatively to whatever you select? Is it all just guess-work, or finding out by trial and error?

Happily, there are at least two methods that may help you determine ahead of time which form of treatment may be best for your pet.

Muscle testing

Muscle Testing, also referred to as Muscle Response Testing (MRT) or Applied Kinesiology (AK), is one possible way to determine, ahead of time, if a food, nutritional supplement, medication, or any other form of treatment may agree or disagree with your pet's energy system. It's a method you can use to make it easier to select the right foods or herbal remedies for your pets, even before you purchase those products.

This technique is based on muscular reactions to specific questions, situations, objects or nutritional supplements. It's already being taught in chiropractic schools and used by a number of mainstream health care practitioners as well.

MRT is a way to read the body by feeling a response from the muscles. It's been said that muscle testing takes the guesswork out of "what to treat" and "how to treat" by allowing the body to reveal precisely where the problem is and what it needs to heal itself.

Most of us have had the experience of feeding our pets something that just didn't agree with them. Their bodies let us know, after the fact, that something wasn't right by producing symptoms of indigestion, burping, excessive gas, tummy aches, or diarrhea. But the body can tell us, *even ahead of time*, through muscle testing, if a substance is likely to create harmony or generate imbalance.

Muscle testing is based on the principle that *the body knows*. Just as your pet's body "knew" when you fed it something that disagreed with it, it also "knows" which substances *will* agree with it and help to maintain balance and harmony.

In a typical example of muscle testing for humans, the person being tested (the subject) is given an herb, vitamin or supplement to hold in his or her dominant hand (the hand used regularly). The quantity used for testing can be one herbal leaf, one pill or the whole bottle of a product.

The subject extends his or her other arm out to the side, level with the shoulder, palm facing down. The person doing the testing (the facilitator) puts four fingers of one hand on top of the wrist of the extended arm, and puts the other hand on the opposite shoulder of the subject to facilitate balance. The facilitator then applies light to moderate pressure downward on the subject's wrist using only finger pressure.

If the substance being tested is something beneficial, the subject will be able to resist the downward pressure and hold the arm rigid. If it's something the subject doesn't need, or something that's not beneficial, the arm will not easily resist the pressure and will drop. It may be only a very slight drop, or it may be a drop all the way down to the subject's side.

If the response is weak—the arm is easily pushed down—the answer is *"No"* (the subject does not need the herb). If the response is strong, and the arm easily resists the downward pressure, the answer is *"Yes"* (the subject does need the herb).

Whenever possible, the testing should be done by the facilitator directly on the subject. However, there are times when you may need a surrogate to help with the testing process.

A surrogate—a person who stands between the subject and the facilitator—is a substitute person who can be used to access information from those who cannot be tested themselves. This might be a baby, a person in a coma, or an animal. The surrogate acts as a clear conduit to transmit the information as long as he or she remains in physical contact with the subject.

It's also possible to use MRT when the facilitator and/or the surrogate are not in physical contact with the subject, but this is an advanced technique which we won't be covering in this book.

Muscle testing a pet

When you have the help of a surrogate, you'll be able to use muscle testing to pre-test the use of foods, herbs and nutritional supplements, or any other healing modality you may want to use for your pet.

To test how your pet may react to a substance using this method, you'll need the products you want to test, the help of a friend or family member, and your pet. The person who is emotionally closest to the animal should act as the surrogate, while the other person will act as the facilitator.

We'll assume for the moment that you're the one who'll be the surrogate. You should spiritually connect with your pet and mentally ask him to allow you to be his conduit for the test. Placing your hand on your pet may help you do this more easily. Remain clearly focused on the animal and allow no distractions. Proceed only when you feel centered and also sense a connection with your pet.

If you're working with a small animal, you may be on your knees on the floor. It's not necessary to stand up. Or, depending on his size, you can place your pet on a sofa, a chair, a bed or a table so you can work at a more comfortable height.

When you're ready to begin, hold the substance to be tested in your dominant hand and touch your pet with the substance. Hold your other arm out to the side, palm down and level with your shoulder. Be sure your body feels as if it's in a balanced position. The facilitator should then use the pressure of four fingers above the wrist of your extended arm to determine the response to whatever substance you're now holding next to your pet.

If the herb, food, vitamin, mineral, nutritional supplement, etc., is not needed by the animal, your arm will go down when the facilitator presses just above the wrist. If your arm response feels somewhat weak and less able to resist the pressure, it's an indication that the product is probably not beneficial for your pet. However, if your extended arm continues to feel strong and resists the pressure, it's an indication that the pet should benefit from using that particular substance.

If you're testing multiple items, one after the other, you'll probably be more comfortable if you relax your arm in between tests. Just be sure, when you're ready to test again, that your extended arm is straight out and level with your shoulder, and that your posture is balanced.

If you don't already have the actual substance, or at least a small sample of it that you can hold in your hand, then write the name of the substance you want to test on a piece of paper and hold the paper in your dominant hand touching your pet. At the same time, hold the clear intention in your mind of testing that particular product. It may also be appropriate to write down as much other specific information about the substance as you can, such as the exact brand name and dosage strength, if that's applicable.

In addition to testing any products or substances you may want to use, you can also put your hand in various places on your pet's body to try to determine if there's a problem with a specific organ, gland, point of apparent pain or infection, etc. As before, if your extended arm easily resists the downward pressure, this is an indication that the point you're testing is apparently okay. If the arm feels weak and drops down, even slightly, this is an indication that there may be a problem or weakness of some kind at the point you're testing.

Testing using a pendulum

There's also another method that can be used if you don't have someone available to act as a facilitator. This method has both scientific and spiritual foundations.

Just as we use a radio to amplify the unseen energy of radio waves so that we can hear music, news broadcasts, talk shows, etc., we can use a pendulum to amplify the response of our own energy field to the energy vibrations that come from any substance we may want to test.

Pendulums have been used for centuries like a form of biofeedback to detect illnesses. They've also been used for some very important scientific and military purposes by people whose names are familiar to most of us. These include Leonardo da Vinci, artist and inventor; Albert Einstein, the renowned physicist; and U.S. Army General, George Patton.

The pendulum doesn't have any inherent powers of its own, and it's not producing any responses; it's only displaying them. It's simply a tool that's used to amplify a person's sensitive reaction to people, places, thoughts and things. What it does is to help you focus your own attention so that you can obtain information from the intuitive side of your brain without a lot of distraction from the rational thinking side of your brain.

The science of Radiesthesia

There's even a science called Radiesthesia that uses a pendulum as its primary tool.

This science has been used successfully to diagnose medical conditions, to measure compatibility (for example, between or among foods, medicines, etc.), and to measure the bioenergetic fields of people. It's also been used to find the locations of landmines, to find errors in computer code, to detect errors in engineering drawings, and in many other significant applications.

Radiesthesia has its roots in a Latin word that means sensitivity to radiation. However, the expression that's probably more meaningful to us in our current culture would be sensitivity to energy or vibration.

But what exactly is Radiesthesia? It's the science that uses a person's sensitivity to the energy vibrations which are coming from objects around them. It's used to obtain information from those levels of energy that we can't detect with our five senses.

How does it work? The science of Radiesthesia uses a pendulum to measure even the smallest vibrational interactions between the energy field of the person doing the testing and the energy field of the object or substance being tested.

This science has been classified into two different forms.

One form, called Physical Radiesthesia, or Microvibrational Physics, can be explained by the laws of physics. It's based on the principle that everything in nature, without exception, is a vibration of energy. The pendulum is the instrument which is used to detect these vibrations. The subconscious mind of the person does not play a central role in Physical Radiesthesia.

In the other form, called Mental Radiesthesia, the person's subconscious reaction, intuition, or "sixth sense" does play a primary role in determining the responses which can be observed through the actions of a pendulum.

Which technique to use?

You can use either approach to do the testing you'd like to do for your pet because the techniques for using either Physical or Mental Radiesthesia are essentially the same. However, since my experience has always involved my intuitive ability, you'll find that the explanation I'm going to provide about the techniques for using a pendulum will be expressed in more metaphysical terms.

You'll be using your pendulum in this sense to amplify your access to your own Higher Self, and through your Higher Self, you'll then be able to connect with the energy of your pet's spirit and the energy of the substance you want to test. That's because the energy of Spirit (God) is always flowing through and around you, your pet, and every object in creation.

Your pet's energy system will detect the subtle energy vibrations of the test items, and this reaction will be transmitted to your own energy system whenever you're acting as a surrogate. The response of these natural energy vibrations will then be transmitted to your muscles, and these subtle reactions will be displayed through the motion of the pendulum.

More about pendulums

A pendulum can be as simple as a chain, or a piece of non-woven thread, preferably nylon, with any kind of weighted object at the end of it. The weight may come in any number of different shapes like a tear drop, a ball, a cone, or a spiral. The material may be brass, ceramic, copper, wood or crystal.

Usually the thread or chain is about eight inches in length, with a knot at the top to hold onto. The length should be adjusted to your comfort level, and it may need to be changed over time. In the beginning, you may find that longer is better, but when you're more experienced, you may want to use a shorter length.

Since a pendulum only displays a response by acting as an amplifying tool, you aren't programming the pendulum to do anything by itself when you're identifying what "yes," "no," and "neutral" answers look like. Instead, your muscles are receiving a message from your subconscious mind. The energy of that message travels through your hand and fingers to the thread. Even though that energy is so subtle that it can't be perceived by your five senses, you can see it being displayed as the pendulum moves in response.

When you're testing something for your pet, your pet's energy field is able to experience the energy coming from whatever that substance is, and it can also recognize whether or not that particular substance will bring about balance and harmony, be neutral or be detrimental.

Your subconscious mind, acting as a surrogate for your pet, then receives that information. But since your subconscious mind can't convey this information to you through any of your five senses, it sends its energetic impressions to your muscles instead, and even the visually imperceptible movement in your muscles can then be displayed through the movement of the pendulum at the end of a thread or chain.

A pendulum should only be used to ask important questions about you, or those you love, and it should always be used only for a legitimate and serious purpose. It's not meant to be used in these applications to predict the future; it should only be used to understand information about things that already exist.

You need to be totally present in the moment at the time you use it for the results to be accurate. Being present in the moment is the same as being in a focused, meditative or prayerful state of mind.

Practical things to know before using a pendulum

Both the subject and the person holding the pendulum should remove any jewelry, watches, or crystals before beginning. For some pets, this means removing their collars.

Before you use a pendulum to test your pet's response to the various substances you want to use, you first need to become familiar with its actions.

Normally, if the answer to a question is "yes," the pendulum will move in a clockwise direction. If the answer to the same question is "no," it will move counter-clockwise.

However, you may find that, for yourself, a back and forth motion means "yes" while a side-to-side motion means "no" (or vice versa), and a circular motion is "neutral" or indicates no answer.

Just like anything else, learning to work with a pendulum requires an investment of time and practice.

Testing the action of your pendulum

Here's a method you can use to test the action of your pendulum.

On a piece of blank paper, draw a circle with a dot in the center of it. Sit comfortably at a table or desk. Place your feet flat on the floor and rest your elbows on the table. Hold the pendulum by the top of the thread or chain between your thumb and index fingers so that it's over the dot in the center of the circle on the paper. Let your other hand rest, palm down, on the table. Be sure that your body is straight, your mind is focused, and that your energy is flowing freely. Allow the pendulum to come to a complete stop.

Relax, and let your breath flow gently in and out. Hold your pendulum over the point on the center of the circle and ask your own energy system: "What does a "yes" answer look like?" Allow the pendulum to start moving back and forth, side-to-side, or in a circular motion naturally. Many times it will start by moving around in either a clockwise or counter clockwise direction. Once you've established how it responds for a "yes" answer, bring the pendulum to a complete stop, then ask, "What does a "no" answer look like?"

Be patient and allow the pendulum to move. It can only move back and forth, side-to-side, or in a circle. Practice several times for at least a week.

Once you have determined your "yes" and "no" answers, you'll need to re-check them periodically. It's not impossible that they may change because of something going on within you, or because of the person or animal you're working with. Simply ask to see again what a "yes" and a "no" response look like at the current time.

Asking test questions

When you feel confident that you know what your "yes" and "no" answers look like, then test them with simple questions or statements for which you already know the answers. My name is . . . My dog's breed is . . . My dog's color is . . . I live at (a specific address) . . . I'm wearing a shirt that's (a specific color) . . . I'm standing up . . . My dog is outside . . . etc.

Ask the question or make the statement in two different ways so that one time the answer should be "yes" and the other time the answer should be "no."

Be sure to phrase your questions or statements using only positive words. Avoid using words like "not," " isn't," etc. For example, if you have a black dog, say either "My dog's fur is black" (to test the "yes" answer) or "My dog's fur is white" (to test the "no" answer).

Testing items for your pet

Once you're comfortable recognizing your own "yes" and "no" responses for questions to which you already know the answers, you're then ready to use your pendulum to help find answers to your questions about the items you want to use for your pet.

Remember to let yourself be fully in the present moment, and ask your Higher Self to be the bridge to understanding your pet's needs. At first, you may not know if you can trust the answers you receive, but with practice, you will develop a sense of confidence.

Place the food, herb, nutritional supplement, or any other item you're going to be testing, on a convenient surface—a table, a desk, a coffee table or even on the floor if you're going to be sitting there beside your pet. If necessary, use a block of wood or an empty box to elevate the item to a comfortable height.

You're going to be acting as a surrogate, so focus on your pet and mentally ask him to allow you to be his conduit for the test. Remain clearly focused on the animal and allow no distractions. Proceed only when you feel centered and connected with your pet.

Hold the pendulum between your thumb and index finger with your elbow slightly bent at your side. Use the hand that feels most comfortable for you. Relax and stay focused.

You may place your other hand on your pet's body if doing so helps you to remain more focused, though this isn't a requirement. Hold the pendulum directly over the item to be tested and ask the question: Is (name of item) beneficial for my pet? Or make the statement: (name of item) is beneficial for my pet.

Remember you should always ask a complete question or make a full statement that requires only a "yes" or a "no" answer, and the question or statement should not contain any negatives.

How you word each question or statement is very important. Your words must clearly express your exact intention. It's not enough to simply ask, "Is this ok?" because sometimes, two things are going on at the same time. At the moment, 1) you may be touching your pet's body and 2) you want to know if the substance is beneficial for your pet to take. If you only ask, "Is this ok?" and the answer is "yes," the response from your subconscious mind could mean "Yes, it's ok for you to touch your pet's body."

You can test the response to your first question by asking the question the opposite way, and by asking other confirming questions, or turning them into statements. For example:

Questions:

- Is (name of item) harmful for my pet?
- Is (name of item) helpful for my pet?
- Does my pet need (name of item)?
- Is (name of item) a neutral substance for my pet?
- Should my pet take (name of item)?
- Can I safely give my pet (name of item)?

Statements:

- (Name of item) is harmful for my pet.
- (Name of item) is helpful for my pet.
- My pet needs (name of item).
- (Name of item) is a neutral substance for my pet.
- My pet will benefit by taking (name of item).
- I can safely give (name of item) to my pet.

If you want to check the response to your first question in yet another way, ask for example, "Is it correct that (the name of the item being tested) is beneficial for my pet?" or "Is it correct that I should avoid giving (the name of the item being tested) to my pet?

If you feel you just aren't receiving accurate answers, even though your questions are properly worded, then it's best to stop and try again at a later time. Possibly, at the moment, you're too worried or emotionally distressed over your pet's condition to remain as objective and focused as you need to be. Some time away from testing may allow you to re-center yourself so that you can then test effectively.

Spiritual protection

Many people like to use specific intentions to assure that they're using their pendulums with the right intention.

To do this, begin by holding your pendulum still. See yourself protected in the golden-white light of divine love. Form each of the following intentions (silently or out loud) and be sure you receive a "yes" response to each statement:

- The response I see displayed by my pendulum must always be guided only by the goodness and love of Spirit (God).
- The answers I obtain when using my pendulum are based only in Truth.
- My pendulum may give a "yes" or "no" response only if my question is clearly stated.
- My pendulum may give a "yes" or "no" response only if the true answer is known, and if it applies to this present time and place.
- My pendulum must remain still or give the "no answer" response if the question is not clear, or if the true answer is not known.

If you receive any "no" responses, consider the cleanliness of your pendulum, and note whether or not your state of mind is calm and clearly focused. You might also try revising any of the above statements so that the wording is more comfortable for you, but still maintains the essence of the statement.

Some important tips about pendulums

- Cleanse your pendulum in salt water overnight (1 tsp of salt in 8 ounces of distilled or spring water). Do this when you first purchase it, and once a month thereafter.
- Keep the pendulum with you as much as possible during the first three weeks while it's absorbing and becoming attuned to your energy.
- Since your pendulum does become attuned to your own personal energy, it shouldn't be handled by others who may impart their energy vibrations to it and thereby reduce its reliability.
- Before you begin using your pendulum each time, have a clear intention in your mind of what you want to accomplish and why.
- Have a list of questions prepared which can easily be answered by a "yes," "no," or "neutral" response.
- Empty your mind of both doubts and preconceptions about the outcome of your questions.
- Ask simple questions at first which will help build your trust in the answers.
- When you're testing items, be sure your questions or statements are clearly and completely expressed using only positive words.
- "Clear" the energy from the pendulum after each question by simply lowering the tip to your hand or to another surface for a moment so that it stops moving. This signals that your question has been answered and you're now ready for the next question. Use this technique frequently.
- It's important to let the natural energy vibrations move through your hand and fingers down the string to the pendulum.
- Some people get better results by holding the pendulum about one inch above the open palm of their opposite hand. This "opens" your energy circuits by creating a bio-feedback loop so that your energy will flow more freely.
- If your pendulum doesn't move very well for you, try opening and closing your hands a few times to activate the hand energy centers (the hand chakras).

- If you're very tired or emotionally distressed, you need to rest and release the emotional distress before you may be able to perceive accurate answers to your questions or statements.
- You may find that you often get the most accurate results when you're helping others.
- Keep a notebook handy to write down your questions and the responses you receive using your pendulum.

* * *

Using either Muscle Response Testing or a pendulum, you should now be able to pre-test almost anything you'd like to use for your pet. Just remember, each time you want to test using either method, you need to relax your mind and body first, and then declare your intention to do the testing on behalf of your pet.

Dedication: In Loving Memory

Chop Chop, one of my beloved Shih-Tzu friends, taught me many important lessons throughout the 14 wonderful years we spent together.

As I was writing this series of books, he taught me one final lesson which I'd like to share with you—the lesson of letting go.

Even with all of my research and knowledge, and despite all of the possibilities for healing that my writings and daily practice contains, I wasn't able to offer him even one more day of quality life.

I realized that when the time does come, sometimes it descends on us so swiftly that we don't have the opportunity to use any healing methods at all. We simply have to accept the fact that it's time for our pets to leave, and the most loving thing we can do is to let them go.

Chop Chop seemed to be doing fine, or so I thought. Then one day he was gone. All I could think was, " . . . but he was fine yesterday, he was fine last week. What happened?"

I was preparing to leave for a book tour in South America and wanted to make sure Chop Chop had enough medicine to last while I was away, so I called my vet and asked for a prescription refill. However, a year had passed since his last blood test, so the vet suggested I bring him in for routine tests just to be sure nothing else needed attention prior to my trip.

On Monday, the urine test came back with satisfactory results, but the blood tests showed fairly high levels of calcium. The vet told me that this could mean any number of things, including kidney trouble or even a tumor. We arranged for an appointment on Tuesday to take some x-rays.

Those pictures revealed that Chop Chop had many stones in both of his kidneys, and about twenty stones clustered in his bladder. Five of them were ready to pass through the urinary tract. On closer inspection of the x-rays, we could see three stones already embedded in the urethra, but they couldn't be passed on through because of their size. If they weren't removed surgically, he would die within a few days.

After the x-rays were taken, Chop Chop seemed to stop being his brave self any longer. It was almost as if he was saying, "Well, now you know, and I don't have to continue putting up a brave front."

For the remainder of that day, I observed that he wasn't able to rest easily, he had a problem lying down, and he'd frequently move from place to place, obviously trying to find somewhere comfortable to settle down. By Tuesday night he was moaning, and he wasn't able to "find a spot" when we went for our walk.

On Tuesday he also stopped eating, although he'd always been the kind of dog who'd lived for food and treats. He stopped sleeping too, where previously he'd slept 20 hours a day. But Tuesday night, nobody slept, even though his discomfort was somewhat relieved with heavy pain medication.

I wanted a second opinion about his condition, so on Wednesday morning, we drove the distance to see my favorite vet and friend, Dr. Sigdestad. Dr. Sig, as I call him, clearly laid out our options.

Chop Chop could undergo surgery on his urethra, an operation that would last about 2 hours. But because he was just one month short of his 14th birthday, and because so many stones would still be in his kidneys and bladder, chances of a satisfactory recovery were very slim. The recuperation time would take about a month, maybe longer, and he would need special care, and a special diet for the rest of his life, which might or might not keep more stones from forming.

I knew immediately that having him undergo surgery of that nature was not the loving thing to do for him. I was going to be leaving for five weeks, and even though he'd still have plenty of loving care and attention at home, I also knew that both the physical and emotional toll he'd have to go through would make it much too difficult for him to endure such an ordeal with any quality of life.

At that moment, it became very clear to me. I finally had to make one of the hardest decisions of my life, but it was a decision I'd promised him long ago that, if necessary, I'd make for him when the time came.

Yes, it did happen quickly—almost too quickly for me to even fully realize right away that his condition was terminal—and definitely too fast to use any alternative healing therapies in one last effort to save his life.

His departure was swift, but he wanted it that way. I know it was his final gift to me to leave quickly, without lingering, and without giving me false hope. I know the timing was right. And I'm certain that it was what he wanted. I'd told him many times that I wouldn't let him suffer, and he trusted me. He had faith in me, and I couldn't let him down when he was clearly ready to go.

Yes, sometimes my heart still aches for the loss of my precious friend, but I have healed. He taught me that it's important for us to let go when it's time, and he taught me to always find joy in living life fully. I couldn't have asked for a better teacher from whom to learn these two very important lessons.

In loving memory, this book is dedicated to you, my FRIEND and TEACHER!

⌘

CHOP CHOP

3/17/92 – 2/22/06

⌘

Epilogue

The series, *For Pet's Sake, Do Something!*, fulfills my dream of writing three books designed to help you come to the aid of your pets whenever they're faced with various distresses or health challenges.

The first book of this series, *How To Communicate With Your Pets and Help Them Heal*, introduces you to the importance of intuition and the art of meditation, teaches you how to carry on a conversation with your pets by using picture telepathy, and introduces you to a number of spiritual and energetic healing methods, plus guided meditations, which you can use for the benefit of your pets.

This book, *How To Heal Your Sick, Overfed, and Bored Pets with Nutrition, Herbs, Supplements and Exercise*, has provided you with a wealth of ideas about how to use fresh whole natural foods, vitamins, minerals, herbs, other nutritional supplements and exercise. These can enable you to improve the overall health of your pets, or even to help them recover from some serious health challenges. This book has also provided recipes designed for pets with special needs, recipes for herbal remedies, and lists of foods all pets should avoid.

Watch for the third book of the series, *How To Heal Your Pets Using Alternative Therapies*. It will offer you information about a variety of alternative healing methods including the use of homeopathy, flower essences, incense, essential oils, crystals, color, sound, massage, magnets, hydrotherapy, acupressure, acupuncture and chiropractic. There will also be chapters about how dogs age; what you need to have in an emergency kit; what you need to know about some emergency first aid procedures; and how to provide for your pet's future if something unexpected happens to you.

Ever since my own dog, Chop Chop, clearly told me I needed to *"Do something"* when he first lay dying at the age of two, I've wanted to share with as many people as possible the many successful methods I've discovered along the way. Completing these three books is a special part of my Life Assignment, and it gives me great joy to know that you, too, are now empowered to *"Do something"* for your own beloved pets!

About the Author

Monica Diedrich knew she could hear animals speak ever since she was eight years old. By the time she was 18, she had also begun to share the gift of her insight and guidance with humans, helping them with their life challenges, as well. Since 1990, however, her work has been devoted *exclusively* to the well being of animals.

She holds the degree of Doctor of Metaphysics and is an ordained minister. Studying Eastern traditions developed her understanding of the natural interconnection between humans and animals as well as demonstrating the importance of attaining healing at all three levels—physically, emotionally and spiritually.

In addition to providing both introductory and private consultations, Dr. Monica presents seminars, teaches classes, and writes books about the art of animal communication. She's also a regular contributor to several TV shows, including one aired in South Korea.

Her first book, **What Animals Tell Me**, has won two awards: the 2001 National Self-Published Book Awards from Writer's Digest; and the 2003 Nonfiction Award, Farmer's Market Online "Direct from the Author Book Award," first place. It has also been translated and released in several other languages, among them, Spanish, Japanese and Croatian.

Her second book, **Pets Have Feelings Too!** was an award winning finalist in the Animals/Pets:General category of the USA Booknews Best Books 2006 National Awards and was listed on USABookNews.com for five months.

In this "how to" series, **"For Pet's Sake, Do Something!,"** she's already completed the first two books and is currently working on the third and final volume.

A native of Argentina, Dr. Monica has lived in Southern California for over 35 years with her husband and children, both human and pet. She can be reached through her website at: http://www.petcommunicator.com.

www.ingramcontent.com/pod-product-compliance
Lightning Source LLC
Chambersburg PA
CBHW070948250726
48663CB00002B/135